"In an age where it is easy to think of ourselves as socially aware and compassionate, but where studies show we are swiftly losing our empathy and growing ever-more distant from one another, this book is a beautiful and passionate call back to becoming fully human, learning to listen to one another's stories and being willing to risk the loss of comfort to live in solidarity with others. . . . Not everyone has a mentor to sit down with for coffee; for those who don't, you will be delighted to find Belinda a wise, experienced, and gentle guide leading you into the high places of true Christian spirituality. I can't recommend it highly enough."

Ken Wytsma, author of *Pursuing Justice* and *The Myth of Equality*

"In *Brave Souls*, Belinda Bauman makes a vitally important and rarely explored connection between bravery and *empathy*. She leads us from conflict zones in the Congo to her own spiritual struggle regarding the universal Christian act of worship and uncovers the stunning truth: only those courageous enough to dive into the depths of empathy will be able to change this hurting world. A masterful storyteller and experienced spiritual guide, Bauman introduces us to some of the most inspiring people we'll ever meet and then invites us—like them and like her—to be brave."

Zach Hoag, author of *The Light Is Winning*

"Belinda Bauman gives us a gift—inviting us away from merely hearing someone to embracing empathy and allowing another person's story to move us into action. The journey isn't pretty or easy, but Bauman's belief in change left me more hopeful than I've been in a long time."

Kathy Khang, speaker, activist, and author of *Raise Your Voice: Why We Stay Silent and How to Speak Up*

"When Belinda Bauman's heart awoke to the suffering of others, she came alive in a way she'd not lived before. On this unlikely journey she discovered that learning and practicing empathy changes the world and changes the one willing to embrace it. In these pages Belinda is inviting you and me not just to feel empathy but to embody it. *Brave Souls* is challenging me to take big risks to love more, and I believe it will do the same for you. Say yes. You won't regret it."

Jamie D. Aten, founder and executive director of the Humanitarian Disaster Institute at Wheaton College, author of *A Walking Disaster*

"Belinda Bauman is a brave soul and her call to live an empathetic life is not just one she writes about but one she's living. This collection of stories, practices, and spiritual truths are words we need to hear, but even more they offer a way of living we need to embrace."

Todd Deatherage, executive director and cofounder, The Telos Group

"Bauman's authenticity, wild stories, and gift with words pulls you into the inner world of a woman being asked by God to listen—*really listen*—to the people around her, specifically to the stories of women who have survived the violence of war. She reminds us—*challenges us*—that empathy is not reserved for a few select saints. It is gritty, personal, concrete, and practical, and available to all brave souls thirsty enough to pursue real love."

Shayne Moore, author of *Refuse to Do Nothing*

"Belinda Bauman tucks 'brave' into the creases of her real life. From climbing actual mountains to diving into the depths of others' stories with care and humility, she has much to teach us about carrying empathy with us, calling it out into the world with our own inner courage. As a leader, mother, and wife, she's inspired me to be more brave in my own life and ministry—and I cannot wait for readers of *Brave Souls* to discover both the risk and the beauty of what it means to live out the fullness of 'brave'! With Belinda as our guide, the journey is worth it."

Ashlee Eiland, midweek director and teacher, Willow Creek Community Church

"*Brave Souls* is winsome in its storytelling and impactful in its truth. In 2016, I spent almost a week traipsing behind Belinda as we climbed Mount Kilimanjaro, and following her lead again through *Brave Souls* only cements my view of her as a visionary and a compassionate leader whose goal is to change the world. With this book, she just might."

Joy Beth Smith, author of *Party of One*

"This is a time for followers of Jesus to 'take heart' in the face of profound challenges, and my friend Belinda has written a book that will help us do just that. Belinda's commitment to justice is grounded in her love of God and her love for people, and her love is one that will inspire anyone who reads *Brave Souls* to follow Jesus with courage."

Michael Wear, author of *Reclaiming Hope*

"This book is the beat of my heart. Belinda Bauman has given us a road map to conquer the biggest mountain in our world at the moment—the distance between us and our 'other.' How do we see the humanity in each other? . . . I read this book with tears literally streaming down my face several times. It gave me hope that we can conquer the mountains of apathy and become the people God has created us to be. Oh, how I want to be this kind of brave soul."

Idelette McVicker, founder of *SheLoves Magazine* and Dangerous Women Tribe

"The beauty and power of Christ-like, Spirit-empowered empathy in a world of apathy and antipathy is the missing ingredient in our homes, schools, churches, communities, cities, and the world. This book is a valuable tapestry of the sad—but true—stories of women and their experiences of violence and injustice interwoven with the joyful and hopeful outcome of authentic Christian love and empathy. You will be inspired, encouraged, and equipped in *Brave Souls!*"

Ed Stetzer, Billy Graham Distinguished Chair, Wheaton College

"In *Brave Souls*, Bauman makes a compelling case to shake apathy and open our hearts. With a gracious touch that doesn't hold back from the truth, Bauman challenges us to awaken to the realities of violence in the world. With so much disturbing news, it is tempting to create a cocoon of comfort. But Bauman provides hope, encouragement, and helpful tools so that we can awaken empathy and in doing so perhaps find love. A beautifully crafted book that will feed your heart, mind, and soul!"

Nikki Toyama-Szeto, executive director of Evangelicals for Social Action/The Sider Center

"Belinda weaves the stories of so many brave and fearless women, who are our teachers and leaders, into a rich tapestry where God's grace and power is the redemptive thread. She ultimately points us to the power of building relationships with those who are on the margins of society, where we so often see God redeeming and restoring his beloveds. I'm so grateful for this book and Belinda's ongoing work of education and advocacy. I believe you'll find, as I did, that this book will inform and inspire you to action!"

Jenny Yang, vice president of advocacy and policy for World Relief, and coauthor of *Welcoming the Stranger*

"Belinda does a masterful job of integrating research, experience, and story to help illustrate the transforming power of empathy. This is a book that searches your soul and prepares you to practice the spiritual discipline of empathy. As a pastor, leader, mother, and neighbor it has invited me to new spaces of bravery."

Sandra Maria Van Opstal, author of *The Next Worship*

"*Brave Souls* is written for this time in history. Belinda's call to empathy, woven with the souls of suffering women as well as research from the finest of universities, disrupts our pious Christian language and smugness and transforms us to living and understanding like Jesus. The writing and stories from the heart and experiences of Belinda are compelling and convicting. The reader is given practical application and guidance in understanding and developing empathy. *Brave Souls* can change hearts and history. This is a groundbreaking and prophetic book."

Jo Anne Lyon, ambassador for the Wesleyan Church

BRAVE SOULS

EXPERIENCING THE AUDACIOUS POWER OF EMPATHY

BELINDA BAUMAN

IVP Books

An imprint of InterVarsity Press
Downers Grove, Illinois

InterVarsity Press
P.O. Box 1400, Downers Grove, IL 60515-1426
ivpress.com
email@ivpress.com

InterVarsity Press® is the book-publishing division of InterVarsity Christian Fellowship/USA®, a movement of students and faculty active on campus at hundreds of universities, colleges, and schools of nursing in the United States of America, and a member movement of the International Fellowship of Evangelical Students. For information about local and regional activities, visit intervarsity.org.

Cover design: David Fassett
Interior design: Daniel van Loon
Images: thumbprint: © Michael Burrell / iStock / Getty Images Plus
      colorful fingerprints: © Lisa Stokes / Moment collection / Getty Images
      watercolor paper texture: © Dmytro Synelnychenko / iStock / Getty Images Plus
      watercolor wash background: © andipantz / Digital Vidion Vectors / Getty Images
      dark flames: © CSA Images / Getty Images
      mountain: © Andrew Merry / Moment collection / Getty Images

ISBN 978-0-8308-4566-8 (print)
ISBN 978-0-8308-7043-1 (digital)

Printed in the United States of America ♾

InterVarsity Press is committed to ecological stewardship and to the conservation of natural resources in all our operations. This book was printed using sustainably sourced paper.

Library of Congress Cataloging-in-Publication Data
A catalog record for this book is available from the Library of Congress.

P	23	22	21	20	19	18	17	16	15	14	13	12	11	10	9	8	7	6	5	4	3	2	1
Y	38	37	36	35	34	33	32	31	30	29	28	27	26	25	24	23	22	21	20	19			

For Stephan, Joshua, and Caleb,

who believed me brave.

For my sisters

who live in war,

who showed me brave.

I beg you, take courage; the brave soul can mend even disaster.

CATHERINE THE GREAT

CONTENTS

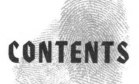

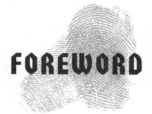

FOREWORD

Christine Caine

Many people enjoy sitting snugly in a warm lodge with a fire burning, sipping hot chocolate while gazing upward at the mountains, and imagining what the view must be like from the top. They love to hear stories about climbers who reached the highest peaks against staggering odds. But few people decide to pay the required price in order to climb to the top and see the sunrise for themselves. Being a spectator often becomes a mediocre substitute for experiencing the real thing.

There is a side of God that can only be known from the top of a mountain, in the middle of a long, hard journey. Standing on this mountaintop, you realize you had more strength, courage, tenacity, determination, resilience, faith, and hope than you ever imagined.

This is the kind of journey that *Brave Souls* is inviting us to join.

It's in this process—the challenge of the climb—that we learn to depend on God for strength to take our next step, even when all we feel is fatigue, frustration, isolation, and hunger. He is faithful to reveal new insights, even when our perspective has become distorted from distraction and exhaustion. When weariness sets in and our vision is clouded, when there seems to be no end to this climb and our minds whisper taunts that our efforts are futile, his Spirit gently leads us onward and upward.

But when you reach the summit and you see the sunrise on a new and glorious morn, it's then you realize that every step—every painful experience, every moment of hardship—is worth the view.

Through making a new journey, the journey has also made a new you. And in this process, God's greatness and goodness in all things is undeniable.

But these mountaintop moments can't last forever. You want to stay here and enjoy the view, the intimacy, but now it is time to go back down. You have had just a glimpse of glory, and now you must go and tell the world what you have seen. It is the mountaintops that give us the vision—a new sight—that we bring with us back down into the valley. This is what we need to see the world differently. And this kind of new sight is what is required to lift the eyes of others and move us *all* to action.

The pages of this book not only contain my friend Belinda's story of her experience but a challenge for us all to see the world differently. I must warn you: this kind of vision—this new sight—will change how you see others and the world around you, *and* it will change how you see yourself. But that's the beauty of it, because this is the kind of transformation our world is desperate for. I highly commend it to you.

A MOTHER'S DAY EPIPHANY

"Shhh! You'll wake up Mom."

It was Mother's Day—*my day*. I woke to the sound of our smoke alarm nearly drowning out the clanking of pans in the kitchen. The pleasant scent of coffee wafted up the stairs, promising all would be well.

Minutes later, my husband, Stephan, and our two sons, Joshua and Caleb, trundled into the bedroom with my breakfast. I sat up to take in the refrains of "Happy Mother's Day!" amid laughter and claims about who made what. Alongside scrambled eggs and sliced avocado, Stephan had slipped in the day's newspaper with this headline: "Congo: The Worst Place in the World to Be a Mother." *I'm always up for being the activist,* I thought. *But this was Mother's Day.* While most of my girlfriends were experiencing Hallmark moments, I was crying into my coffee.

Maybe I had it coming. After all, I had too often reminded Stephan of these words of British abolitionist William Wilberforce: "You may choose to look the other way but you can never again say you didn't know."

God knows my life needed disrupting. That newspaper article explained how mothers in the Democratic Republic of Congo were facing overwhelming odds against raising children in a raging, protracted, unforgiving war. And it became the doorway to one of the most disruptive forces in my life.

I wasn't new to Africa or to activism. For years I'd lived just one country over—Rwanda—and had somehow missed the extent of the suffering in neighboring Congo. The Congolese women I read about that morning were unsung heroes. I didn't just cry; I sobbed. Something deep in my gut told me I had to meet them.

One year later, I found myself sitting on a wooden bench in a rural church near Rutshuru, a town located at the heart of the decades-long conflict, listening to the stories of a group of women. Something significant had led me across an ocean to meet these superhero moms, grandmothers, sisters, and daughters. Their pain-filled stories began a new story in me.

My sisters in China like to say, "When sleeping women wake, mountains move." And oh my, did mountains move for me. There's nothing simple or safe when awakening to your story.

Since that Mother's Day, I've had to fight some pretty daunting odds to tell the powerful and provoking stories of women. At the risk of sounding sentimental, if you're willing to be brave, there's a story waiting to be awakened in you too.

I stake my soul on it.

IF I COULD BE BRAVE

Sheltered White Woman Shocked into Reality After Meeting War Survivor in Congo.

If you are rolling your eyes, thinking, *I've heard that story before,* I wouldn't blame you. I would roll my eyes too, if it were true. But my story was different. Africa wasn't new to me. I had lived in a handful of African countries for nearly a decade by then. I had befriended survivors of war, not just in Africa but also around the world. I had advocated for women's rights and for their stories to be heard. I had served on a hospital ship in West Africa with Stephan, living in and out of conflict zones. Later, when Joshua and Caleb were young, we had moved to post-genocide Rwanda.

But meeting Esperance was different.

Esperance is from Congo, one of the poorest nations in the world, where a woman is subject to sexual violence every sixty seconds. And rape is cheaper than bullets. "You remind me I am still human," she said as she told the story of watching her husband die at the hands of rebels and then being violently raped. She carefully unfolded her sentences as the African sun streamed through the open windows of a cinderblock church. Then we knelt on the dusty concrete floor and prayed.

Somehow, in that moment, Esperance's story became my story. I trust it will become yours too. Her story is raw, and my story is a confession. The lessons we learned together are neither simple nor safe. But I'm more convinced than ever that they contain the power to save us.

After the two of us talked, Esperance asked the person she trusted most, her pastor, to write the words "Tell the world" across a blank sheet of paper. Because she can't read or write, she signed it in the most personal way possible—her thumbprint.

Esperance's Thumbprint: the book you hold bears witness to many brave souls who, like Esperance, did not give up.

WOMEN AS AWAKENERS

By training, I'm an educator. I've taught in state-of-the-art-classrooms, in cinderblock buildings, and under mango trees. I've experienced the joy of watching people move from "I get it" to "I will do something about it." I believe that the best teachers, or at least the ones worth their salt, are awakeners.

Esperance shook me awake. And with her thumbprint, she commissioned me. I added mine to hers, and we launched a grassroots campaign: One Million Thumbprints. The campaign led fourteen others to add their thumbprints to ours, and together they would gather thousands more. Ultimately those fourteen would climb the highest mountain in Africa to "tell the world." And one day we'll present one million thumbprints to Esperance, to heads of state, to the United Nations, and to anyone with the imagination and power to help stop the suffering.

Taking on the issue of violence against women is not just daunting; it's downright terrifying. Women and leaders have been grappling with this issue for years, so I make no claims about my experience or my impact. But I have a mandate, and it's from a woman—a heroine who asked me to lend my voice to hers, to find the courage to join her story, to become a brave soul.

FACING MY OWN MOUNTAIN

But this story isn't just about awakening and advocacy, as important as they are. Along the way, I encountered another mountain that required more bravery than conquering the towering Kilimanjaro. That mountain was me.

> *I encountered another mountain.*
> *That mountain was me.*

While living in post-genocide Rwanda, I saw suffering in some of its worst forms. I also experienced the overcoming of it. Yes, those years changed me, but far less than I thought. I had become more compassionate, more sensitive to the plight of those who suffer. But in my privileged reality, becoming more sensitive hadn't helped me understand suffering and, paradoxically, joy.

To my shame, I was skilled at putting on a pretty good act. I quietly and carefully built a nice Christian wall of protection around my heart that kept others safely distant. It allowed me to avoid too much pain—my own as well as the world's. Somewhere in my journey I settled into high-functioning apathy. I became expert at camouflaging my indifference. I slipped into a season of life when the occasional bursts of clarity and energy for "doing justice" convinced me I was doing just fine. When friends asked about my life, my standard refrain was, "It's all good."

But it wasn't good. I was afraid and restless, and God felt distant. I had developed a strategic numbness that was sophisticated and effective. I had lost my way, and I was afraid of what I had become.

By the time Esperance collided with my world, I was desperate. I wanted to feel again, love again, and be brave again.

I didn't know how.

As I read that article on Mother's Day between sips of coffee mingled with tears, I saw the missing piece clearly. I had forgotten my people. These women who lived in a war zone half a world away, hoping to survive childbirth then praying their children would live past their fifth birthday, were my sisters, my own flesh and blood. They weren't just words on a page or an issue to consider. They were *my people*.

Meeting Esperance and encountering her bravery awakened courage in me to pursue a breakthrough, one I had been desiring for years. I found help in unlikely places—not in the safe confines of my home, or my community, or even my church, but on the front lines, where I met many bold women who were not afraid to confront challenges with grace.

What impacted me most was their capacity to love. They regularly overcame their wounds—physical, emotional, and psychological—and chose to forgive the perpetrators, reconcile with their enemies, and serve their communities. Common to these brave souls was an amazing capacity to empathize, to feel and understand the pain of one another, and to partake in each other's overcoming.

As one trauma counselor put it, "They have learned to suffer well for the sake of joy." This version of empathy was new to me. My version was so watered down it seemed to be nothing more than an idea. Empathy seemed to be full of promise and solution. But when the rubber met the road, it just didn't seem to work.

These women had earned every right to live life as a victim, but they chose to rise above their wounds and do something about their plight. They took the path of empathy, and it was tangible and astonishing. As they healed, empathy became an engine to bring change to their communities. It was real, muscular, disciplined. Its practice drew suffering women out of darkness and into a holy light.

> *Empathy became an engine to bring change to their communities. It was real, muscular, disciplined.*

In short, meeting Esperance and her survivor sisters led me to pursue empathy differently, as a spiritual discipline, making it possible to leaving a clear, healing mark on others while I myself was being healed. My life hasn't been the same since.

EMPATHY ON THE DECLINE

I knew I wasn't alone. Many seem to have forgotten how to understand one another. The University of Michigan conducted a study analyzing levels of empathy in more than fourteen thousand US college students over three decades. The results were alarming: a whopping 75 percent cared significantly *less* about others than the same demographic just thirty years before. Several studies also show that performance in the workplace correlates with empathy. Yet in a most recent study, only 40 percent of "frontline leaders" were considered "proficient or strong" in empathy, with some stating they had "no time for empathy."

In certain pockets of our culture, empathy is an increasingly popular topic; consider empathy marketing, for example. But empathy as a *practice* is declining. Researchers call this the "empathy gap," with some saying it is heading toward extinction.

The consequences of empathy's decline are troubling, to say the least. Indifference—or *apathy*, which literally means "without feeling"—is increasing. One recent headline declared we are in the middle of an apathy epidemic. Outrage is more blatant in our culture as well, and public shaming is on the rise. Americans are more divided along ideological lines than at any point in the past two decades. Political antipathy is deep and protracted.

But our malaise is not limited to politics. In 2015, an NBC poll found that more than half its respondents were much angrier than a year before. Depression, a symptom of apathy, is now considered a pandemic by the World Health Organization, with 5 percent of the global population suffering from the condition. This staggering statistic means one in every twenty people on the planet could be diagnosed as depressed. The saddest part is this: too often people respond with "Yeah, whatever" or "We really don't care that we don't care."

Empathy differs from compassion, at least in the way most of us define *compassion*. Empathy is also a radical departure from sympathy in that it doesn't just involve our emotions. It engages our intellect as well, and it's proven true by our actions. Leaning into the situation, perspective, and feelings of others so we can act for the good of all is a helpful way to understand a practiced, embodied kind of empathy.

Genuine empathy may be in short supply, yet its biological, sociological, and psychological benefits are numerous and proven. Brain studies identify empathy as a key skill that can save your life and the lives of those around you. According to researchers of happiness and human flourishing (what a great job!) at Happify, people who engage empathy are smarter, mentally and physically healthier, recover from illness and injury sooner, have higher self-esteem and trust levels, and live longer. Oh, and let's throw this in for good measure: empathetic people have better love lives. They land more dates and are more likely to marry, stay married, and produce more offspring.

Businesses, educational institutions, think tanks, and economists are looking for ways to increase empathy potential, identify empathy quotients, and develop empathetic marketing. Even diverse faith traditions are beginning to embrace the tools empathy has to offer: empathy art, empathy education, empathy politics, and empathy economics.

EMBODYING EMPATHY

For all the trends, however, embodied empathy remains elusive.

Are you personally experiencing a deficit of empathy? Is your community, whether real or virtual, more polarized than ever? More angry? Is your church split according to political camps? Have you been preparing your kids to stay away from certain topics during extended family gatherings? Is all this leaving you feeling disillusioned or even depressed? Are you struggling to give empathy—to be empathetic—during a time when the world has never needed it more? Or do you find yourself frequently choosing the right mask to put on when you feel precisely—nothing? I have been in that dark place and still have to fight it every day. Together we can figure out where the light is.

Maybe a nagging question sits at the back of your consciousness and rises with each newscast, each self-help trend, each social media post: *What am I missing?* In 2013, the Oxford Dictionary added the acronym FOMO, "fear of missing out." Driven by our desire to self-determine, we check status updates often to make sure we're in the center of it all.

But for all our connectedness, we are subtly—and sometimes not so subtly—ignoring each other's perspectives, circumstances, and needs. Instead of seeking to understand, we quietly pronounce judgment, stoking a simmering anger. Or we smile civilly, nodding our head, feeding the isolation among us.

What are we missing? Maybe we're missing each other. The world has settled for competition instead of compassion, civility instead of love, transaction instead of community. But there is a better way. At the crossroads of your calling and the world's pain stands an age-old something. That something has been tattered and bruised over time, often misunderstood and dismissed. Restored and redeemed, it is a gateway, a portal into recovering our identity within genuine community. That something is what allows us to understand what we're feeling; it allows us to experience joys and sorrows. It listens and learns, is gentle but takes risks, and is kind even as it speaks the truth. And it grows best in holy ground.

We could call it love, but that seems abstract. Too vague. Too loaded. Too many disappointments. If we call it compassion, you may say, "I've tried that, and it didn't work."

Empathy grows best in holy ground.

Empathy needs to be stripped of its baggage and seen anew. In its redeemed form, empathy is a pathway to change—real change. *Holy* empathy is where you and I meet, where we intersect, where we can move beyond superficial love or contrived compassion toward genuine love. Empathy is not an "either you got it or you don't" personality trait, but a skill that can be learned. It isn't a mystical gift or higher state of consciousness. For too long, we've dismissed empathy as irrelevant or contradictory to faith, when in fact it's an essential biblical concept that offers us a gateway to the change we seek.

WHAT'S AHEAD

Esperance's story sparked a new story in me—a journey into the abyss of violence against women, an epidemic far greater and more personal than I'd ever imagined. It is pervasive, yet much of the world doesn't admit it exists, or if they do, they are unwilling to do anything about it. My story has led me through an African war zone, up the tallest freestanding mountain in the world, and into the Middle East. But, above all, Esperance set me on a path that changed me, a journey into the heart of empathy—genuine, audacious empathy, not the fake empathy I'd so often fallen prey to or the flimsy version so often proffered today.

So this book is about a woman from Africa and her impact on me. It's about joining hands to stem violence against women. And, at its core, it's about discovering genuine, disruptive empathy, which is a vision, a commitment, and a spiritual discipline available to each and every person—regardless of temperament, experience, or personality—and a paramount virtue that has the power to save us all.

In part one, we'll look at the inherent power of empathy, including why it's available for everyone, why it has the potential to mend our divisions, and why only real empathy can help us love one another. In part two, we'll explore three skill-based tools for experiencing, embodying, and living out empathy. In part three, we'll discuss how to overcome obstacles to empathy while taking big risks to love more. Woven throughout this book are stories about unlikely people who have done uncommon things in the face of insurmountable odds, including the brave women who live in conflict zones and their sisters around the world.

ONE MORE THOUGHT ABOUT EMPATHY

I realize *empathy* can carry negative connotations. Maybe it's tarnished with personal history for you. Maybe empathy failed you. Maybe it's tucked away in some box of psychobabble on your shelf labeled, "Nice idea. Doesn't work." If that's you, I encourage you to take a risk. Dust off the idea and even the word itself. As you do, you may choose to put an adjective in front of it: genuine empathy, holy empathy, embodied empathy—whatever works for you. I make no apologies for the word. *Empathy* means simply "with (*em*) passion (*pathos*)." It's the opposite of apathy, which means "without passion"—the numb feeling I had settled into before my whole world was disrupted.

> *Empathy is a movement deep in our soul.*
> *It takes us from standing by to standing*
> *up, from sleeping to awakening.*

Empathy is a movement deep in our soul. It takes us from standing by to standing up, from sleeping to awakening. In fact, as you'll see, the laws of God and science say the world must change when we are brave enough to practice empathy with heart, mind, and soul.

So, come now and journey with me. Begin a new story.

Be brave.

PART ONE

WHY EMPATHY CAN SAVE US

He became what we are that we might become what he is.

St. Athanasius

1

BEAUTIFUL COLLISION

You who suffer because you love, love still
more. To die of love, is to live by it.

VICTOR HUGO

I learned about love from a woman named Hope.

Espérance is the French word for "hope," and she and her sisters risked journeying for days by bus, motorcycle, and foot to tell their stories in rebel-occupied Congo. There we sat next to them, women listening to women about their stories of life in the midst of war. We sat for hours hearing the histories of survivors who had witnessed the deaths of their husbands or children, women who had survived brutal rape, torture, and other violence, their pain compounded by rejection from those they loved.

I use the term *survivors* rather than *victims* for this reason: yes, they were victims of corruption, systemic violence, and a soul-stealing culture of rape that had grown up in the weeds of war, but they were not helpless, not voiceless. They were survivors. And with every story, I wondered if I could ever be half as strong as they were.

I remember thinking, *this is Esperance's reality—her world*. When I met her, my eyes took in only the obvious: her orange shirt stained with work. Her pink and blue tie-dyed skirt wrapped around her thin waist. Her white head scarf with a gray bow. Her neon-green flip-flops with white daisies. Her high cheekbones framing her deep-set eyes. Her lips pulled tight as she planted her feet, calloused like the roots of a tree. She was the first of eleven women to speak that day. Eyes downcast, she dutifully told us her name, her age, and the number of children under her care.

Esperance had beautiful hands, although I doubt she thought so. They were dry and rough from hard work, her long fingers elegant, intertwined obediently in front of her as she spoke.

She was fifty. I was forty-five.

She had four children. I had two.

She was a widow. I had no idea what that felt like.

She and I were alike. Yet she and I were so very different.

I was looking at my notes when I heard Esperance say, "You remind me I am still human."

I was looking at my notes when I heard Esperance say, "You remind me I am still human."

I don't recall breathing as she unfolded her story like a new garment, turning back the corners of each sentence: She and her husband had set out to find cooking wood. "It must be done," she said, "even though it's dangerous." Husband and wife met militia soldiers in the bush. Each man carried a machete tucked inside his fatigues, next to his gun. She heard them before she saw them, the click of metal against metal. But there was nowhere to hide.

For a moment, I looked away as she spoke. I was uncomfortable and anxious. I felt cowardly and disrespectful. Taking a breath, I looked at her feet, her hands, and finally her face. She had tears in her eyes. And so did I.

Esperance continued. In a nearby clearing, the soldiers bound her hands. When her husband resisted, she instinctively threw them, still bound, over her head, the universal sign of surrender. She knew all too well what the soldiers would do to anyone who resisted.

First, they shot her husband. Then they flung their fists at her. She was thrown to the ground, stripped of her clothes, and raped. Again and again. Hours later, they left her in the forest, where she remained for three days—torn, bleeding, unable to walk.

As she spoke, she looked at her hands. Her thumbs stroked her thin wrists nervously.

Eventually, she was found by women she now calls "sisters." At the hospital, she struggled through month-long treatments for pregnancy, HIV, and STDs. The rape she'd endured was so violent, so destructive, she said she was "not whole" and could never be fully repaired, even with surgery.

Esperance explained she would have despaired if it were not for pastors who sent her Mama Odele, a trusted caregiver from the church, to her. Pointing to Odele, sitting in our listening circle, Esperance told us how she co-led a trauma recovery program with other volunteer counselors trained and supported by World Relief Congo.

These gentle, heroic women had cleaned Esperance, clothed her, and taken her to the hospital for treatment. When she returned home, they visited her, brought her children food, and helped her find work. Nine months later, these were the women who stayed with her through a complex maze of tears and pain as she gave birth to a baby boy. She finished her story by saying their kindness had brought her back to life. The room was silent as she ended. A holy silence.

TURNING A BLIND EYE

Esperance lives in a country full of beauty, rich with natural resources and an ancient, regal people. The Democratic Republic of Congo (DRC) should be a tourist paradise with its lakes, volcanoes, and mighty silverback gorillas in the vast Virunga National Park. But tourists do not come because Congo is full of conflict. In 2011, a woman as young as three and as old as seventy-three could suffer violence as often as every sixty seconds.

When Lynne Hybels and I first started traveling together to Congo to understand the reasons for the violence and conflict in the region, we found that most of the Western world was turning a blind eye to the problem. Many in our circles had never heard of the war that Esperance lived through every day. These words about the DRC from a 2012 CNN report stole my breath when I first read them:

> The wars in that country have claimed nearly the same number of lives as having a 9/11 every single day for 360 days, the genocide that struck Rwanda in 1994, the ethnic cleansing that overwhelmed Bosnia in the mid-1990s, the genocide that took place in Darfur, the number of people killed in the great tsunami that struck Asia in 2004, and the number of people who died in Hiroshima and Nagasaki—all combined and then doubled.

Yet we rarely heard anything about it. Could it be that pain like this was just too much?

Esperance's words had pierced my soul and left me undone. The ground we tread together felt hallowed. Was her experience heart-crushing? Absolutely. Unjust? Completely. But it wasn't her pain that ambushed me. It was her response to her suffering. Her story—her life—wasn't characterized by the version of love I was trying to live out in my life. Her love was far greater. It was audacious yet sacred, gentle yet fierce, and entirely brave.

I've been obsessed with it ever since.

> *But it wasn't her pain that ambushed me.*
> *It was her response to her suffering.*

LOVE, ACTUALLY

In a café on Fifty-Second Street in New York City, in the fall of 1939, W. H. Auden penned a poem that included one of his most stunning lines in just seven words: "We must love one another or die." There was plenty to fear that year. Germany had invaded Poland, marking the beginning of World War II with its six years of devastation costing an estimated more than sixty million lives. Critics say Auden both loved and hated his poem for a simple reason: his words proved to be true.

With so much pain in our world—personal, global, political, philosophical, and theological—I resonate with Auden. Violence against women had been too much for me to bear, but Esperance gave me a glimpse of hope in one of the most difficult places on the planet. If she could love in the face of so much pain, maybe there is hope for the rest of the world too.

Jesus said, "Greater love has no one than this: to lay down one's life for one's friends" (John 15:13). This kind of love is holy and set apart, the kind that knows fully, that cares deeply, and that is willing to do something despite the cost. But this kind of love is hard to find. When was the last time you were caught off-guard by an unselfish act? Moved to tears by someone's pain? Amazed by the bravery of someone willing to sacrifice for the greater good?

Is it too much to envision this kind of love in our world today? Love in a sea of refugees? Love that convinces people that black lives really do matter? Love for a child who feels different inside than he is on the outside? Love for the person who offended you? Love that knows when to speak and when to act? Love thick and resilient enough to silence disagreement, argument, judgment? Love strong enough to hold back a war and soft enough to open a way for peace?

Even as we've become more connected virtually, we've grown more isolated and distant from each other. More than sixty million Americans—a full 20 percent of the United States—suffer from what sociologists call chronic loneliness. As Mother Teresa said, "The biggest disease today is not leprosy or cancer or tuberculosis, but rather the feeling of being unwanted, uncared for, and deserted by everybody."

> *"The biggest disease today is not leprosy or cancer or tuberculosis, but rather the feeling of being unwanted, uncared for, and deserted by everybody."*
> **MOTHER TERESA**

Had I forgotten how to love—*really love*? It was too easy for me to imagine my enemy as "them" or "those," or anyone against me or different from me, whether across the world, the political aisle, the street, the row of cubicles, or the hallway at church or home. As journalist Susan Faludi aptly wrote, "When the enemy has no face, society will invent one."

For me, it's far too easy to cave in to the lesser angels of my nature, to draw lines, to define who I am by who I am not, unknowingly drinking in complacency as if it were medicine. For me, fear swells. And when I become afraid, everything inside seems to stop. Maybe I justify my caving-in by saying I can't hear. Or maybe I'm too overwhelmed to understand. Or maybe I become too busy to care.

When I stop caring, I stop loving. And when I stop loving, I stop doing. I trade in the messy for the quaint, the gutsy for the tame, the authentic for the fallacious. I give in to pampering. I rationalize apathy. I settle for less. And sadly, I become less.

Something began to gnaw at my soul after I met Esperance. On that holy ground in dusty Rutshuru, she trusted others with her story. And her sisters trusted her with theirs. She knew their stories enough to retell them with their pain, as if they had happened to her. And her sisters could do the same. Those marginalized, vulnerable women regularly laid down their stories for the sake of their sisters.

I wondered, *Have I ever trusted someone like that? Have I ever been trusted to such a degree?*

For the first time in my life, I had serious questions about love and its relationship to faith. My beautiful collision with Esperance left me asking, *What is love, actually?*

THE GOLDEN ROADBLOCK

A law of reciprocity is found in almost every culture. It showed up in ancient oral history as early as 1800 BC. Buddhism teaches, "Hurt not others in ways that you yourself would find hurtful." Confucianism teaches, "What I do not wish men to do to me, I also wish not to do to men." Hinduism teaches, "This is the sum of duty: do not do to others what would cause pain if done to you." From Islam to the Incas, "do not do to others" is a part of each culture's moral code. Even the teachings of Satanism directly state that "to willfully and unjustly encroach upon the freedoms of another is to forgo your own."

Our Christian version of the Golden Rule goes something like this: "Do unto others what you would have them do unto you." It's first mentioned in the book of Leviticus: "Do not seek revenge or bear a grudge against anyone among your people, but love your neighbor as yourself" (Leviticus 19:18). In the New Testament, Jesus said, "In everything, do to others what you would have them do to you, for this sums up the Law and the Prophets" (Matthew 7:12). The apostle Paul alluded also to the Golden Rule in his letter to the Romans (see Romans 2:1-3).

I find it astounding and miraculous and encouraging that cultures throughout history have similar laws of reciprocity. But what happens when the logic in these rules breaks down? "Do unto others what you would have them do unto you" assumes a shared view of what is best. What if what *you* want is *not* what *I* want?

We often try to understand another person through our own experiences. Have you ever shared a vulnerable moment with someone who replied with something like "I know exactly how you feel. I went through something similar"? Did you feel heard? Chances are that reply didn't quite hit the mark, leaving you feeling disconnected and less than understood.

When our listening begins from the point of self—our culture, our socioeconomic status, our privileges or hindrances—we're forced to camp out there for the entire conversation. We aren't really relating to someone else. As well intended as we may be, we are relating only to our own experiences. In Stephen Chbosky's 1999 novel, *The Perks of Being a Wallflower*, a character says, "We accept the love we think we deserve." Hearing others the way you want to be heard means hearing them as if they are you, which they most assuredly are not.

What if the Golden Rule was never meant to be the ultimate standard for social ethics? What if, instead, it was meant to be a common denominator, something everyone could strive for, no matter their background, geography, or faith? In other words, what if the Golden Rule is only a baseline ethic or, at best, a penultimate ethic? It might make more sense to see it through the reverse lens: don't do anything to another person that you don't want done to you.

You may be thinking, *Still, better a world with the Golden Rule than a world without it, right?* It certainly has the potential to make the world more decent. It is a better way to live than with enmity or exclusion. But it is limited—actually, by *us*. How well is the Golden Rule really working for us?

I can't escape an important niggling question: Aren't we supposed to expect more than mutual backscratching, quid pro quo, and tit for tat? To be "done unto" is something every human should expect in their experience. It seems to be the low bar, the on ramp, the low-hanging fruit. Why then do we treat it as something we should *aspire* to when it is merely expected? If the Golden Rule is our aspiration, what the heck is the point of the gospel?

> *If the Golden Rule is our aspiration, what the heck is the point of the gospel?*

MORE THAN GOLDEN

When Jesus said, "A new command I give you. . . . As I have loved you, so you must love one another," (John 13:34) what did he mean? Was he giving an entirely *new* command about love, one that would not just fulfill the law but go much further, something qualitatively better than the Golden Rule? Was he asking us to trade in an interpretation of love limited by our experience, so we can have the transforming power to understand how wide, how long, how high, and how deep the love of God is (Ephesians 3:18)? Jesus described it this way:

> But to you who are listening I say: Love your enemies, do good to those who hate you, bless those who curse you, pray for those who mistreat you. If someone slaps you on one cheek, turn to them the other also. If someone takes your coat, do not withhold your shirt. Give to everyone who asks you, and if anyone takes what belongs to you, do not demand it back. Do to others as you would have them do to you.
>
> If you love those who love you, what credit is that to you? Even sinners love those who love them. And if you do good to those who are good to you, what credit is that to you? Even sinners do that. And if you lend to those from whom you expect repayment, what credit is that to you? Even sinners lend to sinners, expecting to be repaid in full. But love your enemies, do good to them, and lend to them without expecting to get anything back. Then your reward will be great, and you will be children of the Most High, because he is kind to the ungrateful and wicked. Be merciful, just as your Father is merciful. (Luke 6:27-36)

Paul echoed this idea of love at the end of his first letter to the Corinthians as a lead-in to his chapter on love, "I will show you the most excellent way" (1 Corinthians 12:31). This "most excellent way" is a version of love that sacrifices even when not thanked, forgives even when not asked to forgive, defers even when in need, assumes the best even when the worst is assumed by others, treats enemies as friends, and gives away the last penny. This love accepts *what is* before asking what *should be*. This love is a far cry from "do unto me as *you* want done" or even "do unto *me* as I want done."

No, this is a love that says, "Do unto me as my Creator would do. God knows what is best!" This kind of love is rare. Jesus, alive and in the flesh, lived it day to day. He stepped out of his comfort zone, set aside his glory, slipped on human skin, and took up our story to address our deepest need.

Not for the faint of heart, this kind of love.

Still we may think this version of love is reserved for the super-spiritual, the lofty, the better natured, or the saint. But here's the rub: Jesus gave his new command to anyone who claims to *follow him*—not just to his disciples but to anyone who would believe in him through their message (John 17:2). You probably know one or two people who live out this kind of love. Are they saints? Maybe, but maybe not the kind for the history books. In other words, they're probably closer to you and me than we think.

We can't escape Jesus' command "Dear friends, since God so loved us, we also ought to love one another" (1 John 4:11).

So where do we start?

WELCOME TO BRAVE

Meeting Esperance shook my soul awake, leaving me with the weight of one question: *What do I do now?* To my surprise, my answer arrived by email when I returned home from Congo. My friend Larissa was coordinating the hundreds of images, words, and hopes from our time there. Here's what she wrote:

> PS Just received the "release forms" with signatures (or thumbprints where they couldn't write) of the eleven women who shared their stories with you and the team. Belinda— these hit me hard. Even more than any of the stories I read— or perhaps, they rounded out the words—but seeing the

signatures, the fingerprints, seemed to make it all so personal. Even more so . . . their names:

Rachel

Clementine

Fazila

Esperance

Nane

Goreti . . .

Sadly, I've felt slightly cold and hardened as I read the experiences of the women you all interviewed in Congo. But in the last week, I've read so many articles on war, so many statistics on violence, and the numbers feel overwhelming. Numbing.

Then I receive this email. Your women sat with their pastors and people they trust, discussing what it meant for them to sign the release form. Esperance's release form written by her Congolese pastor at her command says, "Go ahead, tell the world my story."

Her permission to tell her story of being raped in the woods.

Sitting alone in my cubicle—it's all too much of a paradox. It's hard not to make it about me—oh, I'm so overwhelmed, I'm so tempted to ignore all this—the pain I feel for them. My pain.

No.

Their pain. Their rape. Their story. Their thumbprints. Their names. I can't do a disservice to them by saying, "It's too hard for me to bear." Those words in themselves are laughable.

Larissa

Larissa was right. I had been home from Congo long enough to know how people sometimes react to the words *rape, sexual violence*, and *rebel soldiers*. Some cough and change the subject. Others shake their heads and click their tongue, saying, "Terrible,

terrible," while they move on to the coffee bar. I understand; it was difficult for me as well. But I knew too much to turn away from my feelings of discomfort.

As I sat looking at Esperance's thumbprint, embracing the truth of her story, I realized how often I had excused my own self from the tension of another person's story. How easily I passed over their pain at the first twinge in my soul. How quickly cynicism and doubt became my default. When had numbness become a viable option for me? The truth of Flannery O'Connor's words came rushing to mind: "The truth does not change according to our ability to stomach it."

> **"The truth does not change according to our ability to stomach it."**
> **FLANNERY O'CONNOR**

I'm ashamed to say that my first response to Esperance's request to "tell the world" was cold and harsh. I thought, *The world won't care.* But "tell the world" burrowed into my soul. I couldn't let that phrase go. For months I carried her thumbprint image with me everywhere I went—her thumbprint stamped under those three words. She had chosen to give her story of pain and redemption away for the sake of her sisters. She had not been undone by her battles but was all the more convinced of the friendship of God through the love of others. She fought to stop the violence around her. Her weapons of choice were not anger or hatred, or even a cry for justice. They were forgiveness and love.

I wanted the violence to stop, but justice was the only weapon for me. Esperance's love was so extravagant, it seemed reckless. For me, stripping away the illusion of a nice, painless, unmarked life meant that I needed to feel the weight of love as it is: pain, suffering, and overcoming. My soul would have to grow brave enough to see each person I meet as C. S. Lewis did: "the holiest object presented to [my] senses." I would need to shed my ability to pay attention or not pay attention, care or not care, as a privileged person. If O'Connor and Lewis and Larissa and Esperance were all telling the truth, caring about others went way beyond being nice and way beyond pain alleviation. These were new rules. I didn't want to just hear someone's story, but to genuinely enter it. Real love looks a lot like having skin in the game.

Real love looks a lot like having skin in the game.

For the first time in a long time, I was willing to take a risk. But I needed to start somewhere. So often action—doing something, even small—is where understanding begins. For me, it meant committing to telling Esperance's story. As I did, a path emerged.

THE ROAD TO EMPATHY

My soul began a slow and steady awakening. It was like wiping the sleep out of my eyes. The hope I found isn't unique to me but is for anyone exhausted by pretense, fear, and saccharin versions of love—even "Christian" love. It's for those brave enough to believe— and live—a better way. However, there was a breakthrough behind the breakthrough. For me, the idea of love had been so abstract, so hard to wrestle to the ground, so hard to *do*. Love felt tinny, hollow, slightly cheap. Jesus' command to love as he loved seemed out of reach for me. Esperance was my example, but I struggled with what it meant for me. I needed a way to understand this skin-in-the-game kind of love.

My breakthrough emerged slowly, over months—and I'm still breaking through. For me the turning point involved re-understanding love as *empathy*—not the nice I'll-do-you-like-I-do-me kind of empathy I had grown up with, which was spoon-fed in school to keep the peace and learned at work so I could manipulate my teammates into doing what I wanted. No, the kind of empathy I discovered is entirely different. It has the potential to revolutionize love, to make it real, genuine—a kind of empathy that converts our talk into action. Empathy, I learned, is the key to Jesus' new commandment, a rule of love that holds greater potential than any rule of gold.

What I discovered wasn't what I'd expected. Empathy is not reserved for a few saints who walk above the earth. It's not a feeling or an epiphany. No, empathy is gritty, personal, concrete, and practical, available for anyone thirsty enough to pursue real love.

> *Empathy is gritty, personal, concrete, and practical, available for anyone thirsty enough to pursue real love.*

This kind of empathy—*holy* empathy—has the power to save us; I am sure of it. It was Esperance's love that ambushed me; it was her empathy that pointed the way, from a simple thumbprint to the towering summit of Kilimanjaro. Two very different places. One destination. It required a road map for me to get there—and the journey between the two made all the difference.

2

THE POWER OF EMPATHY

*We all have empathy. We may not have
enough courage to display it.*

MAYA ANGELOU

"Morning to you, Mama!" The words floated into my tent like a song. It was still dark. Tempted to grumble and roll over to hit the snooze button, I realized where I was. The rough volcanic rock I could feel through my sleeping mat reminded me. Tent. Africa. Mountain.

In one deft movement, a hand unzipped my tent, reached in, grabbed my big toe, and wiggled it vigorously. "How did you sleep? Are you awake? What would you like this morning, Mama, tea or coffee?" After rubbing my eyes, I propped myself up on one elbow and looking squarely into the broad smile of my climbing guide, Ricardo. The African dawn was rising in vibrant gold behind him.

My beautiful collision with Esperance two years earlier had not been just a hit and run. She was the reason I was climbing Mount Kilimanjaro. And I wasn't alone. Fourteen other dedicated "mamas" and "sisters" were climbing too. Guided by the courage to face the realities of women living in war, I had asked women from a wide range of backgrounds to dedicate a year of their life to grappling with the issues of gender-based violence in conflict zones. Some were friends. Some were brave souls I had just met. But each took up the challenge and found their way to Kilimanjaro.

Yes, our guides did deliver hot coffee or tea to our tents each morning. But don't judge us. This little act of seeming luxury served a bigger purpose. The caffeine and sugar injection awakened our oxygen-deprived, elevation-addled brains before we could make the mistake of moving too fast, causing dizziness—or worse, sustained vertigo. Our morning ritual gave each guide a welcome, nonclinical way to check in on us after a night's rest. They hung diligently onto our big toes until we sat up and gave them a coherent answer to all their questions. What seemed like an unnecessary extravagance—steaming drinks delivered to our tent before we got out of our sleeping bags—became a symbol of much more.

"*Jambo sana,*" I croaked with a half-smile. "Coffee please." My voice didn't seem to be working.

It had been quite a while since I'd seen a sunrise. Back home, I was often up at the appropriate time. But stopping long enough to see the actual rising? Not so much. That day I leaned back against my oversized duffel, sipping rich black coffee, letting the mug warm my hands.

A friend of mine had once described my life as marked by holy discontent. I thought maybe she was right. I was a teacher, wife, coach, and mom, but Stephan and I were also ordained ministers, writing and teaching regularly on topics of social justice, prayer, and lament. We had lived in some of the most difficult places on the planet: Benin, Guinea, Madagascar, post-apartheid South Africa, and post-genocide Rwanda.

We knew too much. After years of watching churches and organizations paint people living in the margins as victims in need of rescue by Westerners, we started an organization to work with communities to become agents of their own transformation—heroes among their people—from whom we could learn and with whom we might even become family.

Esperance had left her mark on me like a potter pressing into clay. Her story of suffering was matched only by her example of bravery. She was brave because she wasn't afraid to love—to *radically* love her sisters and also her abusers. I wanted to be brave like her; I wanted to love like her. For me, discovering—or better, rediscovering—the power of empathy would become the pathway to that kind of love.

> *Esperance had left her mark on me like a potter pressing into clay. Her story of suffering was matched only by her example of bravery.*

Sipping the last of my coffee, I sighed. The sun was full, and it was time for me to let the light into some dark places.

This mountain was not going to climb itself.

MY ILLUSION

At the time I met Esperance, I had been experiencing disillusionment at levels I had not known before. Being disillusioned is hard work; remaining disillusioned is exhausting. Everything inside me wanted to cling to a dream that I had been sold and that I had bought willingly:

- Good Christians are nice people.

- God loves nice people.

- God will never give me more than I can handle.

- God wants me to be happy.

Harmless enough, right? But in Congo through the stories I encountered there, the polish seemed to wear off. I knew that God had given me sisters as my teachers, my examples. I was to listen, learn, and emulate. I felt the sting of tears as I thought about the truth,

They were not nice; they were forgiving.

They were not happy; they were at peace.

They had unquestionably been given more than they could handle, which made them brave—very brave.

After years of being a Christian—including years of serving in tough places overseas, leading Bible studies, teaching in classrooms, and facilitating prayer meetings—my fulfilled, happy life was not what I thought it was. My faith was not what I thought it was either. This realization was painful and confusing in the light of my devotion to service, to people. I was experiencing a crisis that hit hard at the core of my identity. "Nice, happy, and protected" were once easy pills to swallow, no matter where I lived or served. Now it all seemed like a double-cross.

"I think the pursuit of happiness is the pursuit of reality," teacher Parker Palmer once said, "because illusion never leaves us ultimately happy." Acknowledging my identity as a daughter loved by God exposed my contradicting realities. If I was loved, then God loved all others, and I was supposed to love as well. But I did not. Real love is accepting responsibility for others, no matter the pain, pressure, or complexity. Real love is willing to take risks by embracing suffering and by rejoicing in the lives surrounding ours. All lives. But I had cherry-picked my "suffering" and "rejoicing" according to what I felt was best. No wonder life felt weighty and significant. I began to accept the truth for what it was and where it was pointing me.

Overcoming my pervasive illusion would prove, in the end, fatal. But sometimes death is good—very good in my case. Much of what

I thought I knew and cared about, and so much of what I did with my days, needed to die. No matter how thick or thin, naïve or sophisticated my Christian veneer, I was getting in the way of learning how to love. The life I wanted—a truth-telling, risk-taking, peacemaking life—was not possible under the illusion of safety and happiness.

On one front, I had bought into the illusion that I could fashion my identity independent of those around me. I sought to be good, right, and properly Christian all by myself—thank you very much. But in the end, I had exchanged compassion for competition and lost my soul in the bargain.

I wasn't alone. Self-determination entices many of us, but leaves us overwhelmingly exasperated, sometimes hopeless. This tribe of independence is growing every day. Our families are smaller, we establish homes farther from each other, and we choose to live alone. We like our space.

On another front, I liked the illusion of being liked. But my flavor of liking looked more like a group air hug than substantive relationships. Twitter and Instagram are initially satisfying for the soul seeking to connect. You can throw thoughts out into this virtual community and, within the hour, fish out a meaty handful of support for your musings. *I am not alone*, you think as you try out another version of your thoughts, your hopes, and even other versions of yourself, endeavoring to satisfy the need to connect.

> *You can throw thoughts out into this virtual community and, within the hour, fish out a meaty handful of supporters for your musings.* **I am not alone,** *you think.*

Until it doesn't.

Sherry Turkle, a professor at Massachusetts Institute of Technology, says virtual empathy can fuel shallowness. Even the most savvy can allow themselves to believe that if they get enough thumbs-ups, they have the equivalent of a friend. Turkle calls this "sipping," adding,

> We are tempted to think that our little "sips" of online connection add up to a big pile of real conversation. . . . Connecting in sips may work for gathering discrete bits of information or for saying, "I am thinking about you." Or even for saying, "I love you." But connecting in sips doesn't work as well when it comes to understanding and knowing one another.

For me the costs were high. Could I recover my birthright, my hardwiring, to love no matter where, when, who, or how? Could I embody genuine empathy?

DKDC—DON'T KNOW, DON'T CARE

When I was a teenager, one of my church leaders had a memorable T-shirt he was fond of wearing to our potluck dinners. Against a black background, white letters spelled this out: "People don't care how much you know until they know how much you care." Today the phrase may be a little threadbare and sentimental, but the idea is ever more salient. To show you know, you have to show you care. Don't attempt one without the other. Practice what is preached. Walk the talk.

A few months ago, I encountered another memorable T-shirt. Its words stopped me in my tracks. I stood, mouth ajar for at least a full minute before my shock and intrigue crashed into each other. Written in black block letters set against a white background were the words "Don't know and don't care," a pithy little unabashed invitation to antipathy.

Stunned and curious, I did what anyone within Wi-Fi range would do. I googled it, and an acronym popped up: "DKDC: acronym meaning, don't know, don't care."

It turns out DKDC is not only fashionable but also a growing fad. At least thirty Facebook pages are dedicated to some version of— you guessed it—DKDC. There you can find thousands of people displaying pride in their self-proclaimed apathy with a flourish. Google again, and you can find hundreds of merchandise options advertising our growing aggressive *whatever*.

Remember the University of Michigan study I mentioned? Remember the alarming results? A whopping 75 percent of fourteen-thousand-plus college students cared less about others than the same demographic thirty years before.

So how in the world had I found fourteen people with enough empathy to climb a mountain to show support for women who suffered in war? Any part of the challenge—the tallest freestanding mountain in the world, the intractability of war, the suffering of innocent women—was enough to put empathy on ice. I had asked each of the fourteen women to give one year of their lives to know and care for others. This was not a walk-in-the-park ask. I had invited them to train physically, fundraise faithfully, toughen up spiritually, read widely, research deeply, and learn diligently about the pain of women in Congo, Syria, and South Sudan, considered three of the most dangerous places to be a woman. I expected them to advocate bravely in newspapers, to talk in front of cameras and audiences and at dinner tables. And, above all, I asked them to conquer a personal mountain in their lives as we climbed Kilimanjaro for others. What they had committed to was far beyond the ever popular "wear a bracelet," "don a T-shirt," or "hold an event." And it was light years away from DKDC.

So why had these faithful fourteen agreed to climb their mountain? One word: *empathy*.

WHAT IS EMPATHY, REALLY?

Empathy is the state of "feeling into" another person's reality. It requires us to find the place in ourselves where we connect with others' experiences, their thought-space, their level of emotions. Researcher and popular author Dr. Brené Brown defines empathy as the ability to join others in their space, essentially telling them they are not alone—in joy or in suffering. Roman Krznaric, a sociologist at Cambridge University, defines empathy as "the art of stepping imaginatively into the shoes of another person, understanding both their feelings and perspective, and using that understanding to guide your actions." This is the place where *I* meets *you*—where souls intersect at the crossroads of love.

> *Empathy is the place where **I** meets **you**—where souls intersect at the crossroads of love.*

Engaging empathy can be painful or joyful, discordant or harmonious. It's almost always full of ambivalence because not only do we bring our own emotions to the space, we also share in the emotions of those with us. As dissonant as this can be, it is the only way empathy works. In order to connect with another person, we have to connect with something in ourselves that knows, at least in part, what she is feeling. To know her pain is to also know her joy; to feel her confusion is to recognize her clarity. Those are the rules. Knowing and caring is a sacrifice for the sake of someone else, and sacrifice always involves risk.

There are two primary scientific camps regarding empathy: some lead with the head and some lead with the heart. And too often, never the twain shall meet. One group views empathy as primarily *cognitive*, the ability to know or understand how the other is thinking and feeling, similar to seeing their point of view. The other group views empathy as primarily *affective*, the ability to feel what the other is thinking and feeling, almost like an emotional contagion. Each view has its own theories, supporters, and detractors. Yet when these two camps clash, we can lose sight of the ultimate goal of empathy.

Thank God, empathy is both—a very soulish kind of space. At creation, God breathed the breath of life and formed humans—not *with* a soul but *into* a soul. A soul is not what we have but what we are: a mind for knowing, a heart for feeling, and a will for acting. Empathy as a way of thinking *and* feeling is the most truthful definition of the brave *soul* God intends for each of us.

But empathy in all its facets is at risk of becoming extinct. Why? Because empathy, at its core, is controversial.

Blame it on Jesus. He came to us as a baby with a body and needs, born in blood and water. Sometimes it's tempting to cede his humanity—that he actually took on our skin—in order to ruminate on his more divine aspects. Sometimes we forget that Jesus temporarily gave up his place beside God to take on the misery and helplessness of those he came to rescue:

> Since therefore the children share in flesh and blood, [Jesus] himself likewise partook of the same things, that through death he might destroy the one who has the power of death, that is, the devil, and deliver all those who through fear of death were subject to lifelong slavery. For surely it is not angels that he helps, but he helps the offspring of Abraham. Therefore he had to be made like his brothers in every respect, so that he might become a merciful and faithful high priest in the service of God, to make propitiation for the sins of the people. For

because he himself has suffered when tempted, he is able to help those who are being tempted. (Hebrews 2:14-18 ESV)

With the arrival of Jesus came the advent of empathy. Jesus became human, one of us—approachable, understanding, listening, and ready to know and care about both our joy and suffering because he was there—fully human, fully aware, fully vulnerable, not distant or removed, but walking among us, giving his life away. The incarnation is the fullest expression of the empathy of God.

Why would Jesus give up heaven, with its joy and peace, for the squalor of Bethlehem, the suffering of Gethsemane, and the torture of Jerusalem? Jesus was—*is*—a brave soul. The incarnation reverberates throughout history as the seismic event that forever links the Son of God with the people he created. It announces the arrival of a "new commandment," the command of Jesus to live a life of empathy with and for others.

Far from simply "walking a mile in our shoes" or "loving us as he wanted to be loved," Jesus chose to know us fully and to care for us deeply—mind, heart, and will—making him our ultimate example.

Consider the opening line of the parable of the good Samaritan, one of Jesus' most famous. "A man was going down from Jerusalem to Jericho, when he was attacked by robbers" is widely accepted as the opening salvo to one of the most compelling stories about empathy in history. It is couched in the context of Jesus sending his followers into the world as "little Christs" with the words "go" and "whomever rejects you rejects me" (Luke 10:16).

The story is a response, actually, to a timeless question by an "expert in the law" (Luke 10:25).

Expert: How do I get eternal life?

Jesus: What does the law say?

Expert: Love the Lord your God with all your heart and with all your soul and with all your strength and with all your mind, and love your neighbor as yourself.

Jesus: Do this and you will live.

Expert: But who is my neighbor? (paraphrased from Luke 10:25-37)

And there it is—every question ever asked rolled up into one enduring and universal conversation: *What matters most in life? What matters most is others.* This is where we as humans always trip up. Even if we know the rules—love God, love yourself, love others—we have trouble with the "others" part. Put a face on the "other," and empathy becomes controversial. The problem is those others are just so *other.*

So Jesus helps us out. He chose to flip the switch with an example of empathy so radical, so real, that it makes loving even the most irritating relative, weird coworker, or scary neighbor a breeze. He went right for the jugular—where the artery of what we know joins with the life blood of what we care about. In this case, "the other" became the hero of Jesus' story.

> "A man was going down from Jerusalem to Jericho, when he was attacked by robbers. They stripped him of his clothes, beat him and went away, leaving him half dead. A priest happened to be going down the same road, and when he saw the man, he passed by on the other side. So too, a Levite, when he came to the place and saw him, passed by on the other side."

Wait for it . . .

> "But a Samaritan . . ." (Luke 10:30-33)

Remember, Jews despised Samaritans so much that they wouldn't even say the name. It's fair to say they dealt more in shades of antipathy. They never expected the hero of the story to be the one they were trying to ignore, to un-see, to do away with. So, pick your poison. What "other" would set you off?

But a . . .

But an immigrant?

But a refugee?

But a Muslim?

But a Democrat?

But an evangelical?

And what about the hero of the story:

> "But a Samaritan, as he traveled, came where the man was; and when he saw him, he took pity on him. He went to him and bandaged his wounds, pouring on oil and wine. Then he put the man on his own donkey, brought him to an inn and took care of him. The next day he took out two denarii and gave them to the innkeeper. 'Look after him,' he said, 'and when I return, I will reimburse you for any extra expense you may have.'
>
> "Which of these three do you think was a neighbor to the man who fell into the hands of robbers?"
>
> The expert in the law replied, "The one who had mercy on him."
> Jesus told him, "Go and do likewise." (Luke 10:33-37)

Likewise to my neighbor. Likewise to the orphan, widow, wandering refugee, evangelical, Muslim, immigrant. Likewise to Esperance. Likewise to you. Likewise to me. Empathy is tantamount to living a likewise life.

BEYOND CIVILITY

Given our turbulent times, rife with racism, sexism, nationalism, prejudice, and bullying, you may feel that empathy is a tall order. Living the way of Jesus—having a likewise life—just seems so lofty. Why not something more possible, something more practical—like civility?

At one time, the Bauman family had the pleasure of living in what is the geographic center of courtesy and decorum. If "nice" had a place, Columbia, Maryland, would be it. We had just moved there when our firstborn—the understated, bone-dry humorist of the family—quipped from our aging SUV's passenger's seat, "Mom, did that guy just cut you off?"

I wish I could say I answered him with measured wisdom, something to guide his emerging character. Something about being patient and kind and understanding, and how everyone bears great burdens. Instead, I think he may have noticed my white-knuckle grip on the wheel, rolling my eyes so hard it hurt, conducting a running commentary about the IQ of the other driver.

"But did you see his bumper sticker, Mom?"

I stopped long enough to read the bright-green sticker on his gleaming bumper: CHOOSE CIVILITY.

Columbia, Maryland, is the birthplace of the Civility Project, brainchild of Johns Hopkins University professor P. I. Forni. In 2006, Forni set out to inspire "gracious goodness" in all of society. Founded on the concepts of respect, empathy, and consideration, the campaign promotes twenty-five rules for a civil society that include paying attention, speaking kindly, being inclusive, and refraining from idle complaints. The initiative is apparently thriving. Hospitals, schools, tourism bureaus, colleges, and even NASA's nearby Goddard Space Center can be found sporting the green Choose Civility logo. The Columbia library alone has proudly given out over sixty-five thousand Choose Civility bumper stickers, just like the one on the car that had just cut me off.

Gathering myself, I apologized to my son for my negative commentary, and he asked, "Mom, what do they mean by *civility*?"

Civility could mean any number of things, so I took my best shot. "I think they want us to be nicer to each other—less aggressive, more tolerant, and, you know, patient." *Good job, Mom*, I thought, congratulating myself half-heartedly.

His response surprised me. "Really? That's it? Be nice? I don't know, it just seems like if we're going to choose something to be, it should be more than just *nice*. And honestly, Mom, I don't know how possible being nice really is." With a sideways glance, he asked, "How do you think civility's working out for the guy in that car?"

Silence.

He was right. You can sport the bumper sticker, but that doesn't make you civil. The painful truth is, civility will never bring real change. It may temper the polarization, emotions, and even some violence. But it will never bring true reconciliation, peace, or love. Even at fifteen, Joshua knew that we need more than civility to rise above the trouble we find ourselves in. G. K. Chesterton suggested we need to raise the bar far beyond civility, declaring that we are "not simply wounded parties that need be compensated, but we are hurt people that need to be healed."

> *Civility may temper the polarization, emotions, and even some violence. But it will never bring true reconciliation, peace, or love.*

TO KNOW AND CARE

I once asked Stephan what I should say when people ask, "What do you do?"

"How 'bout an advocate?" I suggested.

"Nah. Everyone is an advocate of something."

"Activist?"

"Powerful, but maybe a little too powerful," he said with a slight grin. "How about a blogger?"

"Out of the question," I said. I was deep in the throes of the "no one will ever actually want to read my stuff" anxiety that many writers experience. Confidence was not on my side. If I could even get the word *writer* out, the quaver in my voice would certainly betray me.

"How about 'Stephan's wife'?" I asked with a smirk. Always my true north, Stephan groaned. While he loves that I'm his wife, he has always been my never-let-anyone-reduce-you champion. Gently, he suggested I skip to my sweet spot: "You are an educator."

I tried it on. "I am an educator. . . . I like that."

I started teaching twenty-five years ago, and I've experienced the rush of joy at watching people move from understanding to action. My calling is to help others grow into who they are. Of all the things I attempt to do, awakening others is my favorite.

With both science and spirituality pointing to the idea that empathy is part of God's design for humanity, it only makes sense that God wants us to actually *use* it. Taking a page from Jesus' playbook, we could fulfill our mission to live authentic lives if we learn how to handle the hardwiring God gave us.

So, if empathy is pursued by so many people in such a range of disciplines, why does it seem to be disappearing in practice? Maybe because it hurts less when we don't try empathy. Less connection means less pain. Even though we're hardwired to engage empathy, we're also hardwired to avoid pain. The same areas of the brain that control our sense of physical pain switch on when we feel emotional pain as well. Our bodies economize and reroute all pain to a single neural receptor that detects both emotional and physical pain.

In an educational context, empathy is "moving from neither understanding nor caring to both understanding and caring." In essence, it is moving from DKDC to authentic love.

At times I'm keenly aware I was born with deep Jewish roots—like when I can talk only if I can use hand gestures, and I have trouble finding my "indoor voice" when excited. When I was a child, my rural Wisconsin friends would say something shockingly childish, and their moms would say, "Oh my!" But my mom would say, "*Oy vey!*" When we snacked, we *noshed*, and when we complained, we *kvetched*. When we talked of "the war," even in 1990, we were always talking of World War II.

I'm the Christian granddaughter of a Jewish refugee. At age fifteen, Alexis Leon Kolshanov left Wirballen, Lithuania, traveled through Estonia, and boarded a ship for New York. His father had insisted he go for his own safety. Something was politically amiss, and America was the safest place he could think of. But Lady Liberty snubbed Alexis. He was turned away at Ellis Island—perhaps because he was Jewish—but was later admitted for permanent residence in Vermont. He changed his name to Alex Cole, hiding his ethnicity due to the anti-Semitism of the day. The siblings he left behind—my grandaunts and uncles—paid a great price: Alex's brother, Fodor, barely survived Dachau. His sister, Valentina, died at Auschwitz.

As a follower of Jesus, my roots help define me. I still *nosh* and *kvetch*, but my love of the deep meaning found in ancient words has grown beyond the fun of Yiddish. The Word of God takes on beautiful dimensions when I consider what was originally meant. Israel, the home of my ancestors, becomes a place to connect with when considering what it means to suffer with, to care, to know.

Learning among the Jews in Jesus' time required the *will* of the student. *Yada*—or "to know"—is a layered and subtle Hebrew word that means to perceive, to possess, to perform. Learners had to choose the hard work of perceiving, of understanding God's words and his works. The basis for this kind of knowing is profoundly personal, requiring the student to be responsible for—to possess—what they knew.

Educator Geraldine Steensma states, "The [Hebrew] believer was aware that he 'knew' when he lived his commitment, when he exercised his 'knowledge' in every part of his life." In other words, you did not truly know something until you cared enough to let it inform not only what you did with it but who you became. To know meant to care and to care meant to know. They could not be separated. And they aren't dependent on our ability to trust the people we are connecting with. This means we may be hurt or we may be helped. But that isn't the point. Being helped or hurt doesn't dictate whether or not we choose to engage empathy. Genuine empathy is not contingent on the outcome—good, bad, or ugly.

THE WAY OF EMPATHY

Empathy is not a complex tool that will self-destruct if you mishandle it. Neither is it a personality trait, character bent, or rare gift for only a few. Empathy was designed to be used regardless of personality, proclivity, or circumstance. It is custom-made for everyone: business tycoons, high school students, politicians, lawyers, refugees, self-employed mothers, Chinese farmers.

Empathy has an intricate design based in both science and God's word. Behind its complexity lies order, simplicity, even beauty. Empathy not only makes us better at being human but also is key to ensuring our very existence. Without it, we isolate, grow fearful, begin to hate, and ultimately fight. Relationships fall apart. People take revenge. Nations start wars.

Obviously, empathy is distinct from apathy and certainly from antipathy. And what about sympathy? Let's take a close look at each of these "pathies" or ways of relating to others. Imagine you're taking a walk with your coworker at lunchtime. You know each other over conference tables, computer workstations, and a few shared insider jokes, but you don't *really know* each other yet.

Imagine it's a perfect day. The sun is bright, and all is right with the world—except you glance over at your companion and see her lower lip quivering, tears beginning to form. She tries to hide it but then chooses to explain the depth of her problem. In her circumstances, she is sad, scared, and overwhelmed. Your human nature shouts, "Yikes!" and searches for a coping mechanism, a way of feeling, an orientation to the tears so uncomfortably interrupting what was only minutes ago a nice way to walk off that break room cupcake.

Don't be deceived, because you have choices—four of them actually: *antipathy, apathy, sympathy,* or *empathy.* Each has a distinct voice you can learn to recognize. Three of these "pathies" are disconnectors, ensuring a cool distance between you and your teary-eyed coworker. Only one will connect you with her.

What voice will you listen to?

Antipathy says, "I don't know and I don't care." It resists any form of connection with your workmate, clearly communicating no responsibility for her or her circumstances. It chooses intentional ignorance and non-concern. Antipathy simply has no emotional or mental room in this world for anyone outside itself, and may say, "Oh, I just can't listen to your suffering. It's too hard for me to hear." Antipathy suppresses any concern for things we have no direct control over, such as the suffering or pain of others. It is anti-feeling. It takes no risk to care about or to understand the person, perspective, or circumstance. It smacks of arrogance and/or unconcern, and it obviously disconnects you from the person at whom it is directed.

Apathy says, "I know, but I really don't care." Apathy takes on the risk of knowing about an issue but reserves the right to remain at a distance from the responsibility for the issue, leaving behind a mark that is professionally indifferent or judgmental, and undermining any hope for genuine connection. It allows you a superficial connection from a purely objective, aloof, or disinterested standpoint. Apathy can impart a feeling of being diagnosed. It chooses to place value on the facts, figures, and logic of the issue at hand, repelling any sentimentality or emotional concern that may cloud comprehension.

Sympathy says, "I can't possibly know, but I care." It allows you to connect with your companion, but only at an superficial emotional level. It imparts the proper culturally acceptable or visceral response. It chooses to care but limits its level of knowing to only what is necessary, choosing not to get "too involved." It does what is expected to stop your companion from hurting for the moment; it sends a card, gives a hug, tries to paint a silver lining on the situation. Sympathy wears cause wristbands because their friends do. But sympathy can't tell you why or what you must do about the issue. Sympathy takes the risk to care but protects itself from any response that could require connecting further. It's polite civility.

Empathy says, "I know and I care." It allows you to connect with your coworker at an experiential level. Empathy imparts the feeling that you're willing to be with her through it all. The way of empathy chooses to make itself vulnerable by connecting with something deep inside that knows those same feelings of pain, sadness, and fear. Empathy offers action; it fearlessly takes on a problem and moves mountains to help. Empathy takes the responsibility to know what the other is feeling and is marked by compassion and connection. Empathy can actually transform a coworker into a confidant faster than you can say DKDC.

The Four Ways of Relating

SYMPATHY *I can't possibly know, but I care*	EMPATHY *I know and I care*
ANTIPATHY *I don't know and I don't care*	APATHY *I know, but I really don't care*

The way of empathy is most certainly found on the road less traveled, but it isn't hidden. For some empathy is too messy, too connected to relationships, too out of their control. Some feel it's better to ignore the problem so they don't have to care. For others, it's very difficult to believe they can learn to become empathetic. It's easier to believe "I'm just not a very empathetic person." Sympathy is easier—a quick response, an attempt at caring, but without understanding. Often it just makes us feel better but does little for the hurting person.

> *The way of empathy is most certainly found on the road less traveled, but it isn't hidden.*

For many empathy is too fraught with fear, frustration, or the potential to fail. It's much easier to cross to the other side of the road, default to apathy, and continue their journey.

PERMISSION

What we're becoming beckons us to be brave. To learn new ways and pursue love worthy of legacy. W. H. Auden wrote, "All that we are not stares back at what we are." Before meeting Esperance, I sought an identity that I defined for myself, a life that remained comfortably nice and deeply privileged. Esperance's legacy gave me permission to examine my life.

Is this you too? If so, permission granted.

On my journey back from Congo, I found this prayer that has haunted me ever since. It's a well-known Franciscan benediction to be prayed as a blessing. I respectfully call it my Thumbprint Prayer. At first, I prayed it cautiously, since the blessings described in it are a bit daunting. But over time I grew hungry to learn, hungry to know honestly and care deeply. It helped make me brave—brave for truth, for risk, for peace. Brave to become.

God, may You bless me with discomfort,
　with easy answers, half-truths, and superficial
　　relationships,
　so that I may live deep within Your heart.

God, may You bless me with anger
　at injustice, oppression, and exploitation of people,
　so that I may work for justice, freedom, and peace.

God, may You bless me with tears
　to shed for those who suffer pain, rejection, hunger, and war,
　so that I may reach out a hand to comfort them and to
　　turn their pain to joy.

And may You bless me with enough foolishness
　to believe that I can make a difference in this world,
　so that I can do what others claim cannot be done,
　to bring justice and kindness to all our children.

Amen and amen.

3

MAKE YOUR MARK

You cannot help but learn more as you take the world into your hands. Take it up reverently, for it is an old piece of clay, with millions of thumbprints on it.

JOHN UPDIKE

Though there is no consensus regarding how our fingerprints form, the process is known to begin during our tenth week in the womb. One theory is that as the tips of our fingers and thumbs press against our mother's womb, the delicate pressure exerted against the walls of the placenta creates warps, whorls, and swirls into tender tissue, carefully etching patterns into our skin. Though statistically possible, the likelihood of you and another person possessing the same print is one in sixty-four million. No two identical fingerprints have ever been found.

I look at my thumb. The warps and whorls represent my unique identity. Yet my thumbprint also binds me to every other human being that has a thumbprint. When Esperance made her mark, she was giving up a piece of herself in asking the world to care. It was as if her thumbprint was proof she existed—"still human," in her words. I am unique from you, yet you and I and Esperance bear the image of God.

But what about those who live with little love and even less care? And what about the people who wound and disappoint me? Accuse me? Ignore me? They leave thumbprints of a different kind.

We all possess great potential—for good or for bad. We imprint our unique signature on the lives of others.

COSMIC IDENTITY THEFT

My sons refer to the era before social media as antiquity. (Yes, it stings every time.) In less than a decade, social media has restructured the way we view ourselves, others, and the fragile place where the two connect. Referred to as *virtual empathy*, "likes," hearts, retweets, and comments can leave us initially satisfied, but eventually feeling shallow, lonely, and even angry. Social media can keep us from seeing others as belonging to us or as our responsibility. They have the potential to inoculate us from the very thing we need most: authentic relationships. Even the most spiritually savvy social media user can allow himself to believe that if he gets enough thumbs-ups, he has the equivalent of a friend. We also seek "likes" from the people we are closest to, reducing even the people we live with to "liking" us. Are we the victims of cosmic identity theft, selling our birthrights for social media thumbs-up?

I thrived in this space—Instagram, Facebook, Twitter—but was I a "like" junkie? Was I addicted to the quick rush of affirmation in my prefrontal cortex that, if left unmoderated, would eventually damage my soul? I was surprised by how insecure I had become. My identity was woven into my virtual world much more than I was willing to admit.

I gradually began to admit how numb I felt. Did I change my behaviors? Well, no. Condemnation and shame are poor motivators for change. So it seems fitting (and humorous) that God, knowing just how he designed me and where I seemed to be malfunctioning, used social media to snap me awake.

A friend asked me to follow a nonprofit on Facebook that was facing a crisis. While the world was tallying "likes" on its page, what it really needed was flesh-and-blood volunteers. Awareness was certainly part of the organization's values but making a difference could happen only when people showed up and helped. They launched an advertising campaign that included images of refugee mothers holding starving children, a baby amputee, and a girl in a camp, framed by hundreds of thumbs-up emojis to illustrate Facebook "likes." The associated words were haunting: "Liking isn't helping. Be a volunteer. Change a life." The ad won hundreds of awards and increased volunteerism for the organization. They called for brave souls to make a mark instead of just make a "like."

I was their sweet-spot demographic. Their campaign convicted me but also sparked a ray of hope. It showed me a way out of my social media despair. Their elegant solution lifted the bar higher than Golden Rule thinking. It was about real people, real love, and real sweat. I thought maybe my fast-approaching climb up Kilimanjaro would help me break free from my shame. Maybe God was inviting me to shake off my condemnation by giving me an adventure. Maybe God was asking me to breathe in the oxygen of empathy—*holy* empathy—as a source of healing. It was as if there was a guiding hand on my back, and a whisper: "I am with you. Go and do likewise."

And so I did what any self-respecting, recovering social media junkie would do. I emblazoned my hopes on the back of a T-shirt. A local athletic company provided the shirts. A friend created the logo. And we came up with these words:

Tell the truth.

Take a risk.

Make your mark.

Our T-shirts were more than billboards for our collective aspiration. We didn't wear them for "likes." They represented a contract with God, each other, and ourselves to pursue authentic love. God had invited us to do something, and to change along the way. But we needed to admit our insecurity, vulnerability, and self-absorption. Without God and each other, we were a lost cause. With our public declaration, we would no longer turn away from the truth about the world *and* ourselves. We wouldn't shrink back in fear or retreat into insecurity. And we vowed not to cower from seeking the kind of authentic love the world was thirsting for.

AM I GOOD ENOUGH?

Make no mistake, I knew climbing Kilimanjaro would not be easy. For these soul sisters, climbing Kilimanjaro was an act of solidarity with women who suffer violence, and it was a tangible way to raise awareness for a pressing issue.

But attempting to summit with fourteen women was crazier than we'd thought. The statistics were stacked against us. Our bodies fought against us. Natural laws, like gravity and altitude sickness, conspired against us. "Climbing Kilimanjaro," wrote Lynne one year later, "was the hardest thing I've ever done." But climbing the mountain required us to make hard choices. We had to first overcome ourselves. In the end, we were the biggest challenge, not the mountain.

Let me explain. Alanis Morissette's brilliant song "That I Would Be Good" asks whether she would still be good if all went wrong—if she "got the thumbs down," if she "got and stayed sick," if she "gained ten pounds," or even lost her sanity. There's something in the song that strikes deep in my psyche. If I fail and have nothing to offer, do I still count? Am I still good enough?

It's customary for climbers to form a pact before setting out from base camp. "What happens on the mountain stays on the mountain" is the adage. Make no mistake. Oxygen deprivation, chronic cold fingers and toes, little sleep, and challenging terrain works wonders on your willingness to be a little less than kind.

> *Make no mistake. Oxygen deprivation, chronic cold fingers and toes, little sleep, and challenging terrain works wonders on your willingness to be a little less than kind.*

Sensitivities slither out front and center, fears dance at the surface, anger boils over. People say and do things they later regret. Trust me. For these reasons, I swore in blood—well, not quite in blood—to respect the stories of my fellow climbers. The good, the bad, and even the ugly in these pages is published with permission from my fellow brave souls.

Let me just say I was genuinely worried about each of my sisters at different points along the trail. Take Leia, for example. Late one day, just as we were finishing an acclimatization hike and nervously preparing for our summit that would begin at midnight, she ran into a snag. We were becoming familiar with using oxygen tanks in case we needed them. But the elevation and oxygen hoses aggravated Leia's sinuses to the point of bleeding. Tissue, toilet paper, and wet wipes were all precious on the mountain, so by day four, she—being a master of innovation—was using clean underwear to blow her nose. Constantly.

Leia was the definition of a fighter, but she was falling behind. She sat down to recover, only to get up and walk a hundred or so more steps before sitting down again. Every time I turned back to check on the situation, I became more concerned. I connected with our senior guide, Abraham, and had him check in with her. "Leia, would you like me to cry with you?" Abraham asked as he sat next to her on the rocks, reminding her crying makes snot, and snot was not what she needed right now. He could tell she was thinking about giving up. I too could see it in her eyes.

Then Tosha arrived. The oldest of our Tanzanian guides, he had summited Kilimanjaro more than three hundred times. Tosha's gentle, firm manner communicated authority. He was quick to laugh, yet when he spoke, we listened.

Placing a hand on her back, Tosha said, "Leia, do you know what my name means?" She shook her head. "I am the twelfth child of twelve children," he said, smiling. "When I was born, my mother named me Tosha. And it means *enough*." Through the pain and mucus, Leia got the joke and managed a smile. Then Tosha turned serious. "Leia, see, I am here with you, and you have everything you need to do this. You have enough. You *are* enough."

Yep, you guessed it: tears. (And more snot too.)

From that moment on, I could not shake the words, "I am with you. You are enough."

I was reminded of a Jewish tale. A rabbi gave a young boy two pieces of paper with a few words written on each. He told the boy to always keep one piece of paper in each of his pockets. When he was feeling as if he was not good enough, he should reach into his left pocket. When he was feeling proud, he should reach into his right. On those days when the boy was on top of the world, and he felt like all things bent to his will, he remembered to reach into his right pocket. The rabbi's words? "You are made from the dust of the earth, and to this dust you will return."

But when the world was against the boy and left him wondering whether he was good enough, he reached into his left pocket and read the rabbi's note: "The God of the heavens made the universe for you."

Made of dust but having infinite value. What a paradox! We are nothing and everything at the same time.

For most of us, the greatest enemy to doing good—genuinely knowing and caring—is simply this: we don't feel worthy.

> *For most of us, the greatest enemy to doing good—genuinely knowing and caring—is simply this: we don't feel worthy.*

We believe we're not smart enough, not beautiful enough, not strong enough, not spiritual enough, not good enough. Why did Catholic Worker Movement founder Dorothy Day say, "Don't call me a saint! I don't want to be dismissed so easily"? Because if she were a saint, the rest of us could get off easy. We could freely leave doing good to those far better than us—more virtuous, more holy, more spiritual, more Dorothy Day.

So we give up before we begin. We choose apathy or sympathy or even antipathy because we just can't believe we're capable of the virtue of empathy. Leave it for the saints; we're not good enough.

But God says we *are* good enough. Our Creator has no illusions about us. He knows every square millimeter of you and me. God knows full well we aren't capable of virtue. We "all have sinned"; we all "fall short" the Bible says (Romans 3:23). But God became like us so we could become like him—all of us, not just Day or Lewis or Pope Francis.

And herein lies the secret: *we are good enough because God is good enough.* Full stop. Just like Tosha was there for Leia, God is there for us. He makes us good when we admit our frailty, our inability, and even our depravity and decide to follow him anyway. Without

God, Leia gives up, the Jewish boy feels worthless, and we don't climb the mountain or help Esperance fight violence. With God, the sky is the blue, the boy changes the world, Leia doubles down, and fourteen women summit their mountain against the odds, each one overcoming themselves along the way.

"Good enough" became our team mantra. We constantly had to choose to slay our demons by believing in a God who loves us as we are, even as he's making us into something more.

MAKING THE DESCENT

Make no mistake, Kilimanjaro was a breakthrough for me. But it was only one of many steps. I'm always tempted to make the mountaintop the place of destiny, but it wasn't and still isn't. Our journey requires a descent. What goes up must come down into the valley, where we put into practice the choices we made during our moments of glory. When I descend by admitting my fear, cowardice, insecurity, and inability, God makes a way—sometimes miraculously. For me, the way of empathy is an adventure every day.

Apathy is easy; empathy is not. Whether it's sophisticated or sarcastic, apathy never brings positive change. Only empathy leaves that kind of a mark.

Apparently I'm not alone in my tendency toward high-functioning apathy. In a 1976 study, a group of Princeton Divinity School students was assigned a topic for delivering a sermon in class. Half of the students were asked to preach from the parable of the good Samaritan, while the others were assigned topics on seminary vocations. After completing a short questionnaire, one at a time the students were told to hurry over to another building to deliver their talks. Here's the kicker: each of them had to pass by a man (an actor who was part of the study), who was hunched over in the alley, visibly in need of help.

Did they stop to help? The results were telling. Less than 40 percent offered any kind of help to the man. There was no correlation between the topic they were speaking on and whether or not they helped the man in need.

What was a primary factor was whether they were in a hurry. If they believed they were already tardy or were going to be, or if they were "deeply absorbed in what they were going to talk about," they were less likely to be "inconvenienced" by stopping.

On a spectrum from self-absorption to active empathy, the determining factor is making a decision: choosing to notice, to pause, and to take in the presence and circumstances of the other; choosing to admit weakness, inability, fears. When we do both, our hardwired mirror neurons kick in to help us make the choice to act, even if it's highly inconvenient or uncomfortable. Choosing to focus on the other, no matter how *other* he is or inconvenient it is, is key.

Empathy requires us to be genuine. It isn't a tactic, gimmick, or formula to follow. And it requires commitment. I knew Esperance was either mine to love or mine to leave. Being inconvenienced, unsettled, or even deeply uncomfortable can be overcome. We all have a choice either to leave a mark of love or pass by on the other side of the road.

"It would seem that Our Lord finds our desires not too strong, but too weak," wrote C. S. Lewis in *The Weight of Glory*. "We are half-hearted creatures . . . who want to go on making mud pies in a slum because we cannot imagine what is meant by the offer of a holiday at the sea. We are far too easily pleased."

So tell the truth. Take a risk. Make your mark. Or don't.

The choice was up to me, to each of those Princeton students, to Esperance, to Dorothy Day, to my fellow climbers. If it's ours to choose, it's yours to choose too.

ENOUGH

There's a reason guides have you begin your attempt to summit Kilimanjaro at midnight. When your summit is long and steep, and your strength is slim, darkness can be a gift. You have no choice but to be reconciled with seeing only as far as the step in front of you.

Hiking into summit base camp the night before, we were greeted by a bright-green sign announcing that the first of three Kilimanjaro summits was only four kilometers away. But it would take five hours to get there. Still, our goal was finally within reach, the aim of all of our workouts, conversations, and fundraisers for the past twelve months.

At 15,430 feet above sea level, your body begins to do some strange things. The lack of oxygen combined with the bitter cold air left us without an appetite (despite burning about seven thousand calories a day). We joked at how our seven layers of clothes hung loose. Dehydration comes more quickly at higher elevations, but drinking more water brought other issues. It was an increasingly hilarious and Herculean task to "send an email," as we called relieving yourself behind a rock or in the bush.

But this was life on our mountain.

At dinner that night, we took turns praying, sharing our hopes and fears with each other. We agreed the first of Kilimanjaro's summits, Gilman's Point, would be our holy place of peace and protest. We would unfurl our banners and pray for the end of violence against women.

Between prayers, we passed an oxygen-level monitor around the table, inserting our index fingers into what looked like a plastic clothespin. This spiffy gadget measured our acclimatization levels, allowing our guides to gauge our capacity for the hours that lay ahead. Some of us were in rough shape; our oxygen levels were low. To summit together as a group, we'd need an act of God. We reckoned with the possible disappointment, embarrassment, and sadness we would feel if we didn't summit together.

None of us slept well. It seemed only minutes had passed when the all-too-familiar hand unzipped my tent and a cheery voice sang, "You up, Mama Belinda?"

Oh yes, every fiber was up. After a flurry of backpacks, camelbacks, oxygen tanks, and tea and biscuits, we sat together in the mess tent, where Abraham and the guides gave us our final instructions:

- Walk slowly, or in Swahili, *poly poly*. It was going to be the slowest three miles you have ever traversed.

- You are enough. You, and only you, are going to have to do the hard work of climbing, persevering, and not giving up. Remember, your guides are here to support you every step of the way. God too.

- Never walk alone. You need others to make it to the summit.

After slipping on our backpacks, oxygen tanks, and water systems, we began our ascent into the darkness—a slow-moving train of headlamps. We were quiet from the start, breathing, stepping, and watching the boots of the person in front of us. Looking down was essential. We were walking on volcanic scree, small skittish rocks that gave way beneath our boots like sand on a beach. All we could do was focus. *Breathe . . . step . . . breathe . . . step.*

I don't know how long it took before I finally looked up. We were clear of all base camp lights, and it felt like God had called out the heavenly host to cheer us on. Oh the stars—millions and millions of stars! The constellations were as clear as the moon. And if we watched closely, we saw a rocketing meteor or two. Somehow we felt closer to God.

Climbing blind, we couldn't see what surrounded us, but we could feel it beneath our feet. About two hours into our climb, the grade was growing steeper and the scree looser. Another strange thing began to happen: many of us were falling asleep as we hiked. I didn't think such a thing was possible. I asked Kim, our buoyant, Energizer-bunny, abolitionist mama if she was falling asleep. Sure enough, even Kim was, which meant we *all* were. Leia attempted a laugh and said, "I've heard of falling asleep standing up, but this is ridiculous."

Crying out in five-minute intervals, our guides had our backs. Literally. "*Poly poly!*" they implored. "You are enough!" To this we replied, "*poly poly*," or "We are enough," with just enough volume to let them know we were hearing and thinking clearly. At times they also placed their hands on our backs or shoulders to reassure us.

I turned to look back but immediately wished I hadn't. Behind me, I saw narrow switchbacks on a ridge. Gray scree rushed away from my boot like water down a cliff. One missed step, and I would slide for a country mile. I decided I'd better wake up.

Ahead, the trail was bobbing with headlamps. I smiled. I couldn't make out who was who, but I pretty much knew exactly where everyone was. Our resident writer, Joy Beth, our bride-to-be, Chessy, and our marathon runner turned team nurse, Laura, were leading the charge, tall and strong. Our superhumans, Jen and Chelsea, their camera equipment in tow, were catching and recording our not-so-Kodak moments. Kris, our devoted and dry-humored team coordinator, filled out the middle with Kim, Ruth, Brenda, and Leia. Krista, Lynne, and I brought up the rear.

"*Never walk alone!*" rang out. And a chill rolled over me. Someone was missing. We were one headlamp, one voice, one pair of boots, one soul short.

Where was Alyce?

Panicking, I sought out Abraham and shot rapid-fire questions at him: "Where is she? Who was with her? Is she all right?" Abraham had everything under control—except me, of course. "Mama Belinda, she is just there. Look." We turned to look down the mountain to see in the darkness two lights bobbing slowly up the switchbacks.

If you were to ask me what happened that summit morning, I'd recite the facts: Alyce was having real trouble with her gear. She was in severe pain and unable to take the oxygen she needed. Altitude sickness had almost beaten her. She had slowed down, way down. Frank, her guide, was helping her take purposeful steps so as not to give up and encouraging her, albeit in Swinglish, an endearing Swahili/English mash. They had fallen at least a mile behind. We couldn't stop our team to let her catch up. Too much time at altitudes like that could be dangerous. We needed to keep going and pray Alyce would make it.

If you were to ask Alyce what happened that morning, she would say she wasn't just climbing; she was also fighting for her soul. The pain and oxygen deprivation were only secondary to something deeper. In the dark, accompanied by a guide she couldn't understand, she watched as our headlamps grew smaller and smaller in the distance. She began to feel abandoned and afraid. And then the voices came. Voices from the past taunted her, criticizing her for being slow, for falling behind, for not being good enough.

She sat down to compose herself and broke into tears, much to Frank's dismay. She had begun to believe the loudest voice shouting inside her head, the voice of her mother: "You are not an athlete, Alyce. You don't have the build." For the next five hours, echoes of her mother's voice taunted her, goading her to quit, to condemn herself as a failure. But she resolved to take one more step, then one more, finding more strength and hoping against hope the voices weren't true.

Two hours later, I could see the faintest orange outline of Krista in front of me. The sky had begun to turn golden, revealing how far we had come. We laid our packs on boulders and watched the sun rise. Once again, I looked back, searching the switchbacks for signs of Alyce. Her headlamp no longer illuminated the path. My head swam. My heart hurt. I worried she thought we were not thinking of her, not caring.

> *I looked back, searching the switchbacks for signs of Alyce. Her headlamp no longer illuminated the path.*

Lynne and I sat quietly, shoulder to shoulder, taking in the light, letting our eyes adjust to the shifting perspective. The sunrise scattered gold everywhere, bathing the bleak and barren view with light, giving me hope. I looked up at the mountain we still had left to conquer. My buoyed heart sank as I thought about how it would take two hours, at least. Our progress had been excruciatingly slow. I turned to Lynne and said, "What do you think?" When I need brave, she can breathe it into me with just a look.

A smile passed her lips as she said, "Honestly, it looks like Mordor, Frodo." She was right, and turning, the hobbit in me quipped, "I'm glad to be with you, Sam, at the end of all things." After a round of labored laughter at our trading of quotes from The Lord of the Rings, we stood up to climb again.

My thoughts flitted between *poly poly* and Alyce. As I climbed, I decided that a breathing-in, breathing-out prayer was the best use of my time: "Father" on the intake and "help my sisters" on the exhale. Interchanging "my sisters," "my mothers," "my daughters," "my friends," and "Alyce," I wrapped my hope for them into those phrases.

It was almost by accident we realized we could see the top. The path had become very steep. Ricardo pointed out a wrought-iron cross that marked the summit. We could barely see it, but it was there. Just below the summit, volcanic scree gave way to a field of boulders.

Helping each other, one by one, we ascended our last rock. We had reached that peak's summit. Then there was relief, hugs, then photos and awkward smiles, our faces swollen with altitude and frozen with chill.

As we unfurled our thumbprint banners to the wind, I looked for my missing friend, Alyce. Abraham said she was still climbing but was far behind. As we took each other's hands to pray for our suffering sisters in war zones, I continued my prayer for Alyce. "Father [inhale], help Alyce know she is enough [exhale]."

Several of our team members went on to the second and third peaks. The rest were content with the first. But I felt something different altogether. We had defied the odds; we had summited against the prevailing statistics—all of us except one. I thought, *Can Alyce still make it?*

God, I prayed, *if she still wants to summit, and the guides say she can make it, I will summit again, with her.* I had barely finished when our guides pointed out the first snowstorm of the winter season moving in quickly. Best to get off the mountain—our full descent to the night's base camp was still eight miles away.

The next hour passed in a blur. Climbing down the boulder field proved to be even harder than climbing up. The team split up into smaller groups, descending at different paces and caring for those who needed help or encouragement. I descended with Lynne. Each meter down, I wondered if Alyce would be able to make it up.

An hour later, having descended the boulder field, someone yelled, "It's Alyce!" My heart leapt. As Ricardo began speaking to Alyce's guide, I searched her eyes. She was exhausted and tearful. But I saw the same fire in her that I'd seen before. "I want to summit," she whispered.

Alyce needed someone to carry her oxygen for her. I wrapped my arms around my sister and said, "Girl, never walk alone!" As we began the ascent, I slid the oxygen tank on my back. Alyce walked close behind me, taking hits of oxygen when she needed it.

We struggled, slowly, *poly poly*, to the top. We stopped and rested often. Two hours later, we set foot together on Gilman's Peak. We held each other and cried.

That day our guide Abraham named Alyce "the Lioness," meaning she was a fierce fighter. Today Alyce wears the word etched in silver around her neck.

REFLECTIONS ON THE SUMMIT

In the Talmud it is written, "We do not see things as they are. We see things as we are." The journey Alyce and I took was complicated and messy, fraught with questions and doubt. On our way down the mountain, Alyce whispered, "I wanted this, Belinda, for the sake of the women and my daughters. I know you wanted it for me. You believed in me and took on my challenge like it was your own. I am enough. We are enough."

When we summited, each of us exchanged a small point of view for God's larger one. We traded our fearful perspective for a fearless one.

As we reflected together, I realized I hadn't once worried whether we would succeed or fail. I didn't fear—for me or for Alyce. Somehow I had managed to take on the pain and joy of another without hesitation, without rationalizing and second-guessing. The hindrances of indifference, apathy, and judgment had fallen away. In that moment, I experienced a freedom I had never known. By summiting with Alyce, I had summited my own mountain. And the view was breathtaking.

I later told Alyce I needed two summits—one alone and one together—to help me understand empathy. When we summited, each of us exchanged a small point of view for God's larger one.

We traded our fearful perspective for a fearless one. It was more than a metaphor, more than an act of solidarity with each other and for the women who climbed. It was physical, yes, and emotional. But it was also spiritual—a spiritual transaction that we would apply to the rest of our lives.

What we saw on the mountain was God's perspective. God wanted us to see who we are in his eyes so we could view others the way he sees them. For a moment, dark had turned into light—enough light to make us want more. An immense struggle gave way to overcoming, a moment of transformation that would continue. Sure, it would ebb and flow, but something fastened to our souls on that mountain.

For me, it was a realization that I could relate more closely with brave souls living out empathy. Our testimony was becoming anchored in something real and timeless, something revealing and healing for us all.

AWAKENED

On June 15, 2014, billionaire philanthropists Bill and Melinda Gates gave the commencement speech at Stanford University. It began normally enough, with thank-yous and congratulations and honors. But near the end, as Melinda Gates leaned into the podium, she said to Stanford's best and brightest, "Here is our appeal to you: as you leave Stanford, take your genius and your optimism and your empathy and go change the world in ways that will make millions of others optimistic as well." Then she lowered her voice and smiled. "You don't have to rush. You have careers to launch, debts to pay, spouses to meet and marry. That's enough for now." And then she turned serious. "But in the course of your lives, without any plan on your part, you'll come to see suffering that will break your heart. When it happens—*and it will happen*—don't turn away from it; turn toward it. That is the moment when change is born."

Around my neck, etched in silver next to the image of a thumbprint, I wear the words *Brave Soul*. For me, these words hold in tension both suffering and joy. It's at the intersection of these two beautiful words where I need to give and be healed.

Is your soul in need? Are you drawn to live a life of "likewise" and claim the courage that comes as you do? Along with Alyce and Abraham, Leia and Tosha, and each of the women and guides who summited Kilimanjaro, I am here to testify that we are enough because God is enough.

PART TWO

LEARNING TO LOVE

I know it may seem small and insignificant, but it's not about what it is, it's about what it can become.

Dr. Seuss, *The Lorax*

4

PERSPECTIVE-TAKING

*I wonder how many people I've looked
at all my life and never seen.*

JOHN STEINBECK

Last year Stephan and I took our sons to Chicago just after Christmas. We walked the Magnificent Mile in the bitter cold. We warmed ourselves with deep-dish pizza at Gino's East. We watched ice-skaters whirl in the falling snow in Millennium Park, and took selfies by the Bean.

One night on our way back to our hotel, a couple approached us, asking gently, even sheepishly, for "some small change." Stephan said hello and asked for their names. "I'm Jennifer," the woman said, her eyes reflecting the Christmas lights illuminating the arctic night. "And this is my husband, James." She was nervous at first, but then explained their plight, pausing often to make sure we were still listening. "We have three kids. They're back under the bridge with friends. . . . James is an electrician. He lost his job. He's trying to find another. . . . When he went to look for a job last week, someone hurt me and . . . well . . . I'm not sure I can try to find a job right now."

"It's okay," I said as she teared up. James looked down.

Stephan offered to take them to a restaurant, but together we decided to help them pick up a few things at a nearby convenience store. We waited near the register while they apologetically combed the aisles. The other customers seemed fearful. Stephan explained quietly to the clerk that we had them covered, so he needn't call security.

Two boxes of cereal, several cartons of pudding, some granola bars, and some soda later, we walked out together, laughing and sharing stories about their kids and ours, their careers and ours. We listened to their ideas for next steps. It turned out Jennifer had hope after all.

We exchanged pleasantries as we parted. Jennifer teared up again, and I did too. And then she said something I will never forget: "Thank you for seeing us."

People tell me all the time they aren't the empathetic type. What they imply is that empathy is only for certain people—those with a specific personality bent, patient temperament, or Samaritan's call. In other words, empathy is a gift for the few, not a mandate for the many.

They are dead wrong. We don't get off that easy. Empathy is a skill that *can be*—and indeed, for the sake of our world, *must be*—learned. And it all begins with perspective-taking.

GAINING PERSPECTIVE

Some years ago, researchers Solomon Asch and H. A. Witkin conducted a series of studies on how people orient themselves. Participants were blindfolded and placed on a chair that had been tilted to a certain degree in a room that was also tilted. Their job was to find the "true upright" position in a room without windows or other markers to give them any clues as to how to orient. The results were fascinating. While some were able to find their upright position, many were off as much thirty-five degrees—yet they thought their position was normal. Why? They lacked a context to orient themselves. They assumed their perspective was right, but they were dead wrong.

Without some means to gauge, we naturally orient ourselves according to what we deem trustworthy from our own perspective, no matter how distorted our perspective is. Awakening to the perspectives of others can radically change how we see the world and how we love others.

If empathy is "the art of stepping imaginatively into the shoes of another person" in order to gain understanding and perspective, then perspective-taking is a secret weapon against apathy, sympathy, and antipathy. Indeed, we cannot love without it.

Sometimes called *theory of mind,* perspective-taking helps us bring out the best in others and stave off a worsening situation. It helps us interpret what others are experiencing in two ways: by opening ourselves up so others can affect us (*empathetic receptivity*) and by seeing others as agents, or "possibilities," who can make choices and take action (*empathetic understanding*). Perspective-taking can help us negotiate, motivate, and activate, and it requires us to be thoughtful and reflective. But key to this process is the need to be truthful with ourselves about our *own perspective* in order to consider another's.

In the story of the good Samaritan, the unlikely hero is surprisingly receptive to the suffering of the traveler in a context where everyone assumed their perspective was right. Jesus painted a backdrop where hatred was the vice du jour. The Jews despised the Samaritans and vice versa. But Good Sam was curious—another empathetic skill important to perspective-taking—as he approached the unconscious man in the middle of the road. The apostle Luke wrote that he "came where the man was" (Luke 10:33). Unlike the priest and Levite before him, the Samaritan made himself vulnerable, even putting himself in danger, while also opening himself to receive.

Kneeling down to the man, the Samaritan would have realized his situation. The man was a fellow traveler, vulnerable just as the Samaritan was. By receiving him as human, the Samaritan found courage to imagine himself in his predicament, perhaps feeling his pain and fear. He interpreted the bruised and bloodied man not as an enemy to be feared but as a neighbor to be loved; he allowed his heart to feel the man's suffering, which moved his hands to act.

He saw. He felt. He acted.

I can still hear Jennifer's words, "Thank you for seeing us." How many times have I not considered another's perspective?

How many times have I played the role of the priest or Levite, perceiving the dark lump in the road not as a fellow traveler in need but as a distress-inducing situation to be avoided or a time-sucking complication to be ignored? Excuses within their cultures led both the priest and the Levite to miss an opportunity to love, to act, and to be changed. Instead a man they would consider an enemy overcame his fear and chose the way of empathy.

> *How many times have I played the role of the priest or Levite, perceiving the dark lump in the road not as a fellow traveler in need but as a distress-inducing situation or a time-sucking complication?*

Perspective-taking almost always involves messiness. Knowing and caring about others means investing in understanding their context, past and present, personal and corporate, as well as their limitations and advantages. Perspective-taking is an embodied experience that helps us see our lives and the lives of others in context.

If we aren't paying attention, we can find ourselves standing at the place where understanding and misunderstanding intersect, the very crossroads where shame can throw us off, skewing our vision of the person right in front of us. Our perspective, like our thumbprint, is both uniquely personal and highly universal. When it's off-kilter, it can affect not only our life but also all the lives around us.

HOW TO SEE THROUGH OTHERS' EYES

Our world suffers because we have an abundance of "my opinion" and a deficit of "I see where you're coming from." Taking the perspective of another is one of the most powerful God-given gifts at our disposal.

Because we can learn, we can change. When we change, we grow braver. "Learning life's lessons is not about making your life perfect," says Elisabeth Kübler-Ross, "but about seeing life as it was meant to be." Risk, love, and empathy are at the heart of each of these lessons, helping us form an understanding God's design for our own soul.

Having learned and relearned many of these lessons, on the mountain and off, over what felt like a long and humbling season, this what I know: a brave soul lives free or dies trying. This is how we know we are becoming brave: our enslaved hearts are set free. We experience freedom from living a stilted, shallow, off-kilter life. Freedom from ignorance, fear, antipathy, and apathy. Freedom from self-centered sympathy, self-concern, self-loathing. And freedom to become ourselves as we open up to those around us—the most profound freedom of all. "Through others, we become ourselves," said psychologist Lev Vygotsky. Paradoxically, shifting our perspective to another's can help us become who we are meant to be.

But perspective-taking is not easy or automatic. It took a woman from Congo to awaken me and a climb up Kilimanjaro to find the courage to live it. Between the two, I began to learn the skill of moving from "my here" to "their there." Even for the brightest mind and most earnest heart, the waters of perspective-taking are fraught with questions and conundrums. Sometimes, people question the questions. But moving from not knowing and not caring to knowing and caring is possible.

Sometimes we feel threatened when we're challenged to take in a view other than our own. Challenges can leave us stuck, even paralyzed. We stop growing. We become restless. We stop loving. I know this well. I was stuck until I found courage to confront the hard truth. When I take someone else's perspective, I sometimes feel I'm giving up my identity, my rights, my opinion. I feel threatened and protective. But Christians should be the least threatened, most open-minded people on the planet. Where God leads, God gives grace.

So, how do we actually move from "our here" to "their there"? Let's start with a road map.

Is there anything more comforting than a map when you're lost? That blue traveling dot on your GPS or that red arrow on the map in a mall brings great tidings of good news: YOU ARE HERE. And once you know where you are, you can see where you want to go.

In their book *Real Influence: Persuade Without Pushing, Gain Without Giving In*, authors Mark Goulston and John Ullmen help us understand perspective-taking. They write that perspective is nothing more than a fixed point from which you view someone or a situation. Perspective-taking means simply assuming *someone else's* fixed point—intellectual, emotional, and/or spiritual—without necessarily giving up your own. Imagine you are on your way to meet a friend at a café. You are at southeast end of the city; he is on the northwest end. When you call him, how will you tell him where to find you? If you say something like "To get to where I am, start in the southeast corner" makes no sense. You are beginning at *your* here, not *his* there. Yet this is often how we try to live with others—on our terms, with our assumptions, from our perspective. We begin from experiences with our point of view. When we do that, we miss the opportunity to connect. "There's a communication chasm between us and them," say Goulston and Ullmen, "but we're acting as if they are already on our side of the gap."

A friend of our family once told us about an experience he had on one of his many long-haul flights. After settling into his seat, he began chatting with his seatmate and discovered that the man was a business owner and a devout Muslim. They talked at length about each of their families, especially their children, who were close to the same age. They connected as dads, as husbands, and as frequent travelers. Midflight, the Muslim father of three joined a few others in the open area of the plane by the bulkhead to pray the Maghrib, or Muslim sunset prayer. Immediately, upon seeing the man kneel to pray, call buttons began going off all over the plane. Nervous passengers notified attendants, worried something sinister was going on.

At that moment, our friend said he felt what it must be like to be a Muslim dad living in a world that distrusts who you are. The time he spent in conversation helped him move from his "here" to the Muslim man's "there."

JUMP THE GAP

I jumped the gap on top of Kilimanjaro. I moved from my perspective to Alyce's and was able to join her in her quest to overcome.

As we came down the mountain, she shared how she had moved from her perspective to mine, believing that she could summit if we did it together.

We all have the raw materials we need to jump the gap. Remember how our mirror neurons are finely tuned to respond to the social information we get from others? Princeton neuroscientist Kimberly Montgomery suggests mirror neurons are actually "engaged selectively to simulate actions that are most informative for understanding the mental states of others." Mirror neurons point to the idea that we were created to be able to see the world through another's eyes. Science, not surprisingly, helps us to live out the design of God.

But how do we engage these natural synapses? When I first met Esperance in the war zone, seeing through her eyes was painful. All I wanted to do was take her away from that situation. I even inquired about relocating her. I could see her situation only from *my* perspective, not hers: Would she want to leave her home? What would she fear? What were her dreams? Where would she go? My good intentions toward Esperance were inspired by altruism but were fueled by my own fear and egoism.

I was functioning from my "here" not her "there."

My good intentions toward Esperance were inspired by altruism but were fueled by my own fear and egoism.

If you were to ask any one of us Kilimanjaro climbers at any point during our journey to the summit, "So, how are you?" you would not have heard, "Feeling super strong! Ready to go again tomorrow!" We knew we were all struggling and why we were struggling. That's why we willingly entered each other's struggle— and how we found courage. Empathy begins by recognizing our weaknesses, which takes bravery. We need God's help to choose. God took our perspective by literally putting on our skin with all its frailties, yet he does not condemn us. And he calls us to approach him for help: "For we do not have a high priest who is unable to empathize with our weaknesses, but we have one who has been tempted in every way, just as we are—yet he did not sin. Let us then approach God's throne of grace with confidence, so that we may receive mercy and find grace to help us in our time of need" (Hebrews 4:15-16).

God himself empathizes with us, so we can empathize with others. Empathy becomes an audacious act of love, securing our divine rights—rights given to us by God from birth—to know and care for others. The fictional good Samaritan raced past the egoist priest, who chose to protect his own "rightness," and also past the altruist Pharisee, who chose to follow the prevailing "rightness" of his society. He was the paragon of a brave soul as he took the perspective of the wounded man on the side of the road, seeking to right the wrong. I like to imagine at that moment, he acted exactly the way his Designer had created him to act. His mirror neurons were synapsing.

WHERE YOU STAND MATTERS

When we start caring about the point of view of others, we realize that asking questions is key: Where are they coming from? What is important to them? Where am I coming from? What is important to me? For example, because I knew about Alyce's background and her great desire to summit, I started to care more about her point of view. Her desire to summit became my desire for her too.

It turns out there is some science to this as well. As you think about the person you're seeking to understand, consider the following three aspects of perspective-taking.

1. *Physical perspective.* These characteristics of a person are easily observable or easily knowable. Where is the person from? What does he do for a living? Where did she grow up? What challenges does he have merely because of his age, gender, color, clothing, or professed faith?

2. *Attributional perspective.* This is our educated guess or hypothesized understanding of another person. I may not know if she is an extrovert or an introvert, the state of her bank account, or her health. Is she hungry or did he recently suffered a traumatic event? Imagination is key to this perspective. You engage your imagination to "read the air" in order to try to understand the person's perspective. Relational histories, socioeconomic status, social cues, and verbal and nonverbal cues all contribute to your hypothesized understanding. One caution, however: attributional perspective-taking is only helpful when we leave judgment and stereotyping out.

3. *Conceptual perspective.* As we recognize there is a gap between "our here" and "their there," we must also remember that our perception is colored by our own state of being. What assumptions do we have to challenge in ourselves to close the gap? Where could we be wrong? Importantly, seeking to understand another person's perspective doesn't need to threaten our own convictions, but does need to correct our assumptions. Understanding is never an act of weakness; instead, it frees us to express love.

THREE ESSENTIAL STEPS TO AWARENESS

Our mountain guides were experts at situational awareness. They were aware of our surroundings, of each climber, of the path we were on, and of themselves. As we watched them, our team learned to become aware, not just of our own issues but also of each other's. Abraham, chief among our guides, was brilliant at finding solutions, aware of the problems each of us faced, and attentive to our skills or limitations as he helped us find our way up.

Increasing our awareness in these three ways—physical, attributional, and conceptual—is helpful for jumping the perspective gap with each other as well as for opening our eyes to God's point of view. Applying the following three-step process has helped me increase my situational awareness and gain increased perspective.

1. Humanize. By asking good questions, gathering information, and listening well (see chapter five), we humanize the one we wish to connect with. When we drop the us-versus-them mentality and signal that we care for the other person as God does, we break through the most significant barrier to empathy: the idea that *some people matter more than others*. Goulston and Ullmen suggest we humanize when we understand another's "strengths, weaknesses, goals, hopes, priorities, needs, limitations, fears, and concerns . . . [and] demonstrate that you're willing to connect with them on a personal level." When you begin to hear things like "You get me" or "Wow, you understand!" you know you're experiencing a breakthrough. Body language—smiles, eye contact, gestures—is also telling.

It's important to remember our own constraints and challenges when working to "get" a person, to love her as she is. Letting her know you see her limitations and constraints without casting judgment or offering opinions creates an environment conducive to understanding one another. Neither Ricardo nor I expected Alyce to move up the mountain at lightning speed, for example. We weren't thrown off when she rested often or when tears came. She was brave within her limitations, and we wanted her to know she was affirmed, not judged, and that she was enough, no matter what.

2. Mind the gap. When we demonstrate our willingness and ability to understand someone's context—his opportunities *and* his challenges—we show we genuinely know and care about his situation. But observing and orienting to his situation requires us to acknowledge our own opportunities and challenges as well. When we do, a gap emerges: the difference between our situation and his. Identifying this gap is essential to perspective-taking.

Use your senses to become aware, to observe. Take in your environment and establish what your normal is for the situation. Ask what's going on. What is the mood? What body language or tone of voice is being used? One of the most important things I did was see that Alyce was missing. As we climbed together, I stopped and observed her, whether from a distance or face to face. Her demeanor, her tone, her movements told me much about how she was doing.

Also use your attributional skills to scan for anomalies—that is, things that should happen but don't or do happen that shouldn't. Is he sitting with arms folded when he is normally open? Is her brow furrowed? Did she take the seat furthest from you, when she normally sits closer? Are there outside distractions? This skill can be practiced in everyday environments and conversations.

3. *Shift your perspective.* When we show people that we understand their context, that we "get" them, we demonstrate empathy and empower change. When we shift our perspective, we're able to consider their personal stakes, offering possibilities for making things better while bringing clarity and reducing anxiety. When you succeed, you'll hear comments like "That could really work!" or "I see how that would help me." This is your opportunity to become their personal empathy advocate.

I'll never forget Alyce's face when I offered to carry her oxygen tank. Once I began to experience the power of perspective-taking, I started to recognize it everywhere, even in some unlikely people like Sarah Silverman. A comedian, actress, and producer, Sarah is usually described as opinionated, vulgar, sarcastic, outrageous, and sacrilegious but very talented. She referred to her work in an interview with Katie Couric as "demented humor." She focuses on social taboos and controversial topics such as racism, sexism, politics, and religion. Needless to say, she uses sarcasm and shock to make her point.

A couple of years ago, I opened my news feed and clicked on one of her YouTube links: "Sarah Silverman Is Visited by Jesus Christ." How could I resist that? Christian clickbait at its best. The video portrays a popcorn-making, movie-binging, hair-braiding Sarah with Jesus. They talk about all the taboos. The video ends with a pitch for her project called "V to Shining V," a campaign for women's reproductive rights.

I penned a Facebook post in response: "Dear Sarah Silverman, I am NOT alright with this. I did not hear a single thing you wanted to say . . . so if that was NOT your goal, I suggest you not alienate, offend, and hurt the people you are trying to speak to."

And so began my journey "against" Sarah Silverman. With just one post, my gavel of judgment had fallen. From my perspective, I knew *this kind* of woman. I did not care for her, and it was *not* okay for her to mock my faith. Ultimately, in the name of Jesus, and to my shame, I took up a serious offense. I never posted again. I never wrote her a letter. I never boycotted, or spoke out against her again. In fact, I barely ever thought of her unless she came up on my radar. My true colors would show in my response along some iteration of "Can't stand that woman!" This went on for a long time.

Until this year.

Audrey Assad, worship leader, writer, and all-around peacemaker, tweeted a story about Silverman with this tagline: "Please don't tell me the love of God is not possible in everyone." She linked to an article titled "Sarah Silverman's Response to a Sexist Tweet Is a Much-Needed Ray of Hope."

As I read, I was ready to have my eyeballs singed out with f-bombs and name-calling. But instead I found myself in tears. As part of her new show, *I Love You, America*, Sarah, a self-described liberal feminist New Yorker, was tweeting about having dinner with a right-wing family from Louisiana. Sarah was asking a genuine, straightforward question about life in Louisiana, when, out of the blue, a man mean-tweeted her a word, a word that, in his perspective, summed her up and dismissed her as a comedian, as a woman, and as a person: "c*nt."

Yet instead of skinning this man alive with her searing, smart, and sarcastic wit—she could have eaten him for lunch—Sarah responded, "I believe in you."

You see, Sarah had taken the time to read through the man's entire Twitter history. Somehow she had mustered up the courage to read his story, slip on his shoes, and feel his pain. (Turns out Sarah experiences back pain just like him.) She continued, "I read ur timeline & I see what ur doing & your rage is thinly veiled pain. But u know that. I know this feeling. Ps My back f***ing sux too. see what happens when u choose love. I see it in you."

In the next five tweet exchanges, he told her he could no longer love due to childhood sexual abuse, his medical history, his drug history, and his poverty, loneliness, and physical pain. With each confession, Sarah showed him he was seen, heard, and cared about. By the end of the exchange, she was asking her Twitter followers for help from any medical doctors in the San Antonio area, and she established a GoFundMe page to help pay for his medical costs.

Sarah took his perspective. As she did, the sexism and hatred faded away. The expletives disappeared from their discourse, and all that remained was two human beings caring for one another. He apologized for his word in his own way. She forgave him in her own way.

The capacity to understand another person's story, to comprehend the subtle backdrop of experiences, both excellent and limiting, is a holy thing.

The capacity to understand another person's story, to comprehend the subtle backdrop of experiences, is a holy thing.

When we transcend our personal narrative to get over ourselves, we become gap-closers, ones who, as Paul said, can approach the throne of God with boldness, asking for ourselves to be put aside so our brave souls can rise to the call (Hebrews 4:16 NIV).

I'll never forget the moment Alyce and I claimed our summit together. Tears streaming, the pain in our legs and lungs screaming, but we felt free. We were enough—not merely good enough, brave enough, or heroic enough. No, we were enough because we boldly accepted God's perspective of us: we were loved as we were, then and now, whether or not we summited.

5

EMPATHETIC LISTENING

The first duty of love is to listen.

PAUL TILLICH

I don't know what I expected.

Mountaintops *should* be noisy places, with wind, weather, and rumbling rocks. Our team had just achieved its goal: summiting the rooftop of Africa for our sisters. I guess I had imagined it more like a Super Bowl touchdown, all whoops and cheers. But we didn't experience any hoopla at all. We experienced something much better.

Kilimanjaro has a 30 percent grade at the summit. Before climbing Africa's rooftop, this meant nothing to me. Now it means crazy steep, and impossibly hard. Each breath comes at a cost. Oxygen rushes in and out, scraping over your throat and nose while your brain focuses on each gasp.

So our conversations with each other ceased as we strained to pull ourselves over the final boulder field to the first of Kilimanjaro's summits. We managed to give encouragement without words, gesturing with our eyes and outstretched hands. As we climbed the last of the terrain to see the iconic Gilman's Peak sign, something powerful enveloped us. Our gasps for oxygen subsiding, we surveyed the magnificent view. We exchanged meaningful glances. A few whispers emerged. Then we listened to the quiet.

It felt like we had entered into the house of God with what little we had—the breath in our lungs, the care we offered each other, the bravery in our souls—bravery transferred to us through the thumbprints of our supporters and suffering sisters. As I stood on the edge of the world, looking down on the miles and miles of steps we'd taken from the bottom to the top, I imagined Elijah hiding in the mountain cave as Jezebel hunted him. He was tempted to despair, to give up. There he listened for the voice of God. It was not in the toppling wind, or the crushing earthquake, or even in the all-consuming fire. Instead, God made his voice still and small (See 1 Kings 19:11-13 NIV).

Divine quiet doesn't mean divine indifference.

Divine quiet doesn't mean divine indifference. How God speaks is as intentional and as important as what he says. And so it was with us. My journey from thumbprint to mountaintop taught me that brave souls listen with audacious empathy.

As a team, we had heard each other's fears and failures. We had listened to each other's testimonies of healing, forgiveness, and overcoming. We had read each other's bodies and minds. Rarely in my fifty years have I felt so cared for, so understood, so listened to as I did in those days.

As we quietly hung our banners filled with thumbprints at the summit, we watched the sun light up the glacier on the other side of the crater. Our breathing became more regular, and we found our voices. We moved in close and our guides joined our circle. Slowly, quietly, Joy Beth and Ruth began to sing the only words in all the world that seemed important at that moment, beckoning us to join our voices with the "voices of many angels, numbering thousands upon thousands and ten thousand times ten thousand" in Revelation 5: "Worthy is the Lamb" (Revelation 5:11-12 NIV).

The mountain had become a holy place. We had cursed it at times, but that day we blessed it. It became sacred, and it remains sacred. We had come to shout from its rooftop, to announce, to proclaim. But we found ourselves listening instead.

DEEP CALLS TO DEEP

If perspective-taking is slipping off our shoes to slip on another's, empathetic listening is walking around in them.

> *If perspective-taking is slipping off our shoes to slip on another's, empathetic listening is walking around in them.*

There is no empathy—no authentic love—without genuine listening. But listening is elusive. And sometimes even suspect. One thing is for sure: in today's noisy world, listening—genuine, empathetic listening—is rare.

The good news is we are hardwired to listen—the first communication skill we encounter in life as babies. We grow into more effective levels of listening, which are far beyond the simple decoding of sounds. When we listen, we grow. We develop. We change.

So why is listening so rare and so difficult? Author and activist Austin Channing Brown wrote these words of encouragement to our team before our climb:

Often when you're weary, when you're tired down to your bones, your body tells you that no one else is experiencing the pain you feel. Conversing is difficult. It's hard to hear the voices of those around you over the throbbing in your knees or the never-ending to-do list running through your head. . . . Not only is your body weary but your capacity for connection is cramping along with your calves. It's hard to serve others when everything hurts, when you have to focus just on the act of breathing. Your brain tells you to love those around you, but your body screams to focus just on yourself.

Life gets in the way of listening. More often than not, we are in a hurry, a hassle, or a hustle. We lose our way, and life wears on. During my years of self-protection, I forgot how to listen to the ones I cherished, those I worked with, and especially those I didn't like. When I tried to listen, indifference kept me from seeking to understand. To my shame, I tuned in only long enough for a break in the action, waiting for a breath between words, so I could jump in with my own thoughts and opinions.

Brave listening requires letting go of yourself to pursue someone else instead. In the silence the mountain, I learned some hard lessons. I learned I can give my ear to those with me and even those opposed to me. I can validate others' thoughts and feelings. I was grieved thinking about my years of nonlistening, when I resorted to sympathy, apathy, and even anger. As I closed my eyes in the stillness of the summit, I whispered, "God, I have not listened. Forgive me."

Someone once said, "Listening is so similar to loving that sometimes you can't tell the difference." Listening, a Jewish adage explains, is done with much more than your ears. Engaging your soul in the spiritual discipline of empathetic listening is tough, but it can help heal this world. We can't love unless we listen.

The human race spends up to 80 percent of its waking hours communicating. We write for about 9 percent of that time, read for around 16 percent. Thirty percent is spent speaking, but a whopping 45 percent is spent listening. Scientists say the vast majority of that 45 percent is done at an ineffective level. What would happen if we were to convert our everyday listening—45 percent of our total daily communication—into empathetic listening? I believe what C. S. Lewis called the "deep magic" would happen, an unrivaled wave of love so powerful that pain is dulled, trauma is healed, body and earth regenerate, and souls long dead are brought back to life. In other words, listening with empathy is a redemptive act.

LISTENING IS LOVE

It was the beginning of rainy season on the border between Rwanda and Congo. I scanned the room for anything more solid than the blue-and-white USAID canvas to keep out the impending deluge. Nothing but two-by-fours and tarp. Then I grappled with my thoughts of the frenetic journey, the condition of the camp, the prolonged suffering of my Rwandan and Congolese sisters. As my sisters told their stories, I was learning to listen to the way they said their children's names, the smiles in between, the tears waiting to fall, the lifted chins when they said the word *survivor*. Poignant periods of silence entered the room as well, bringing healing—the healing of refugees, displaced families, child soldiers, slaves mining gold and tin, and men waging war.

I needed to hear those stories.

I asked fifty-year-old Uwimana Marie how she and her sisters had come to the refugee camp. She was haggard and beautiful; she pulled her sweater close as clouds threatened. "When you are a refugee, you lose everything," she said, her hands moving as she spoke. "But the most painful part is losing your right to think. I used to think about my farm, my goats, and the education of my children." She lifted her head to look into my eyes. "Now I only think about how to survive each day." Four others nodded, and another began to tell her story of loss and lament.

The Nkamira Transit Camp, where these five women lived, was in Rwanda, just over the border from Congo. To say the camp was filled to capacity is an understatement. It had taken a month of requests, letters of intent, and interviews with government agencies before a kind and overworked camp director agreed to arrange a meeting with a group of refugee women between the ages of forty and eighty. He had led me past the tarp walls and tin roofs of the eleven warehouse-sized living blocks. There I met women and children who had fled the violence that has come to characterize the Democratic Republic of Congo. They were living their lives in this place: cooking, washing, carrying bundles of charcoal, kicking a ball made of banana leaves and trash, waiting in endless lines. Every voice I heard seemed to have a quiet hum underneath it: "Can you hear me?"

Refugees were meant to stay a maximum of three days. Uwimana Marie and her four companions had been there for more than nine months. The homes they had fled were miles away, deep in the bush, across a very dangerous border. Congo is known as "the most dangerous place to be a woman," "the worst place to be a mother," "the rape capital of the world," and "the world's greatest humanitarian disaster." The conflict there is regarded by the international community as intractable. Six million are dead, 2.7 million internally are displaced, over half a million are refugees, a woman or child is raped every sixty seconds, and nine out of ten refugee women between the ages of three and seventy-two have experienced gender-based violence. In Congo, mothers often tell their daughters what to do not *if* they are raped but *when*. On all accounts, this is an international crisis of mass proportion, yet so few people know. And if they do know, jumping the chasm to caring enough to listen is usually too big a leap.

In light of these overwhelming odds, what do these women think about? What gives them hope? What do they fear? How do they see God?

Uwimana Marie began speaking again, detailing her flight. She seemed to sit taller as I listened. "My village was attacked at night. We stayed hiding on the farm as long as we could." She leaned toward her companions.

"When the gunfire stops, you check and hope, check and hope. But the gunfire always starts again. Then you know your family must flee with empty arms, without your goats or your friends or sometimes your closest family." Her eyes grew dark as she spoke of her husband and oldest son, who had stayed behind to guard the farm. She had not heard from them since. Her shoulders slumped.

> *"When the gunfire stops, you check and hope, check and hope. But the gunfire always starts again. Then you know your family must flee with empty arms."*
> Uwimana Marie

All five women had heard gunfire and screams through the night. They held the hands of their smallest children, praying their husband or mother or sister was able to lead the older ones. They traveled only at night, using the dark to their advantage in hiding from those who sought to rape them, steal their children, take their lives.

I asked what the women thought about God. As if by some agreed-upon signal, they all sat up straight, squared their shoulders, and boldly said, "*Yego!*" which means *yes* in Kinyarwandan. Nyira, at seventy-six, the oldest of the group and married for "more years than I can remember," said with confidence: "God is certainly here and listening to us as we talk right now! We each reached a place of safety and are still alive. We have shelter and hope that our families may yet come to us. God is here because he hears, and we have hope."

Some women shared how God had blinded the eyes of soldiers and militia men that chased them, allowing them to cross the Rwandan border safely. One was able to find her lost child who had slipped away from her in the chaos and dark. All the women had been surrounded by violence, yet none of them had a debilitating physical injury. The credit, they insisted, went to a God.

They even found God in the meager food supplies in the camp. "When you finally reach a place of safety, then you can eat," said Kamanzi Rosa, a fifty-nine-year-old mother of four. For these brave souls, that meant three to five days of hunger. The women also revealed how keeping a hungry child quiet while pushing forward in the dark is truly an impossible task. I also tried to comprehend just how God comforts a shaken, malnourished refugee with only 3.5 kilos (about eight pounds) of red beans, 12 kilos (about twenty-six pounds) of maize, and pinches of salt and oil—the food they received when they arrived at the camp. Yet they were comforted by the strong belief that when we ask God for bread, he will not give us a stone (see Matthew 7:9).

WE MUST FORGIVE THEM

Each woman spoke forgiveness for those who violated their dignity, thieved their bodies, murdered their family members. Each testified to the power found in forgiveness. "If we forgive those who hunted or hurt us, it is not from us but from God himself," whispered Kamanzi Rose. "If we keep the bitter burden in our hearts, it would destroy us. We must forgive them. We must not wish to kill them as they wished to kill us. Our lives were threatened, but we are still alive, and so we must forgive."

When I asked them what they feared most, the question hung in the air. The response came slowly, resolutely: "We fear being forgotten. . . . There is no hope when you have been forgotten." This is not the kind of forgotten that leaves you off a party guest list or being "unliked" on social media. This is the kind of forgotten that creeps around the edges of the most crowded room and whispers, "No one sees you, and no one cares." When a woman becomes invisible, isolated, abandoned, ignored, and forgotten, even for just a moment, it sinks deep into her soul, leaving fear in its wake.

"When we hear those who hear us, it gives us hope," Nyira said, smiling through her dry lips. "Hope is to know that others know us." I took her hands in mine as she looked at me with her wise eyes.

South Africa's Archbishop Desmond Tutu said, "My humanity is caught up, is inextricably bound up, in yours. We belong in a bundle of life." We cannot live fully if we are isolated, alone, or forgotten. I felt and saw the strength of women who had endured the deepest of suffering and yet hoped in God. Belonging to one another began with listening.

When I returned home, Stephan gently reminded me to, "Honor them as they honored you." Friendship means shouldering burdens and joys together, listening and remembering, even across an ocean and through a war zone. As they say in Rwanda, "Sticks in a bundle are unbreakable." By listening again and again to the stories of women who suffer the pain of war, I try to honor the image of God in each of them. Through not forgetting what I have heard, I honor the holiness of their suffering and bind myself in friendship, placing my thumbprint next to theirs.

DON'T KNOW HOW TO LISTEN?

Empathetic listening does two things: it connects mind and heart to the person speaking, and it seeks to understand before being understood. Connecting with someone can be fraught with misunderstanding and missed connections, especially given the level of noise swirling around us.

The unrivaled listening champion on our Kilimanjaro team was Mama Brenda. Maternal to her core, she had been mentoring young parents and coaching frazzled moms for decades. When I asked her to climb, her husband, Don, encouraged her to take up the call. She said, "I want to let these women know they are not alone, that someone cares for them and their children. I want them to know that there are women on the other side of the world that are willing to help."

In Congo, Brenda kneeled and prayed with obstetric fistula patients—their vaginal walls torn from traumatic birth or violent rape—as they recovered from their fourth, fifth, and sometimes sixth surgery. Her brave soul called out to theirs as she took their hands, sometimes not speaking at all.

As she and I talked, I told her a story about my then five-year-old son, Caleb. I had reminded him at the beginning of each walk, "Wait for Mommy so we can hold hands and cross together." Once after crossing three intersections holding my hand, he started to make a dash at the fourth. With my heart in my throat, I caught his arm and said, "Did you listen to me? Wait for Mommy!" Big, sad eyes and silence followed. For weeks, this process played out, every single time we crossed a road.

One day, after catching his arm as he was trying to dash away, I asked again if he was listening. Tears welled up in his baby blues, and he choked out, "I try. But I don't know how."

The truth hit me like a brick. I had viewed listening as natural, as if all we have to do is flip a switch. All I had to do was remind my boy to listen, and he would magically be able to do it. The truth is, we must learn to listen in order to survive. Unborn children listen to their mother's speech for nine months and are able to distinguish it from others at the moment of birth. As children grow, they use this learning to hone in on the protective guidance of their mother's voice.

> *I asked again if he was listening. Tears welled up in his baby blues, and he choked out, "I try. But I don't know how."*

Conversations today are often like Ping-Pong matches. You serve up an opening sentiment. The other person analyzes the trajectory and hits a zinger back. Whoever is silent first loses. So the essence of much of our communication becomes competition.

Communications researcher Julian Treasure proposes a compelling reason for this: we have grown impatient, taking in our information in soundbites. Memory and careful attention are no longer essential ingredients of communication. Because of this, Treasure points out, "The art of conversation is being replaced by personal broadcasting." In essence, we are all out there talking *at* each other instead of *to* each other. Media outlets shout at us to catch our attention, and we find ways to shout at each other just to be heard. "This is not a trivial problem," laments Treasure, "because listening is our access point to understanding. . . . A world where we don't listen to each other is a very scary world indeed."

Listening is a complex, multilevel skill we are born with; yet it requires development at all ages and stages. As I learned with Caleb, it also requires a great deal of grace. Everyone is telling some kind of story, from the body language in the checkout aisle to the tone of voice at the dinner table. If we listen well to others' voices, their body language, and even their silences, our own body rewards us with a shot of chemical encouragement—a mix of the hormones serotonin and oxytocin—telling us to keep up the good work. Sometimes called the empathy hormones, they promote connection though a willingness to put the welfare of others first. When we actively listen to others, oxytocin promotes trust and feelings of commitment. Serotonin is the molecular manifestation of the feeling we get when we know we've been listened to.

"These little considerations for others have a building effect," according to *New York Times* bestselling author Simon Sinek in an interview about his book *Leaders Eat Last: Why Some Teams Pull Together and Others Don't.* "The daily practice of putting the well-being of others first has a compounding and reciprocal effect in relationships, in friendships, in the way we treat our clients and our colleagues." Empathetic listening is not only good for each of us but also for our community. Scientists believe even small acts of empathetic listening every day provide little shots of serotonin and oxytocin not only to the listener and the listened to, but also to anyone who hears the conversation. What kind of crazy-generous God designed our bodies for such a fantastic return on investment?

In the same generous way, God designed our soul to benefit from empathetic listening too. Brave souls who listen deeply to others are rewarded with increased patience and kindness (1 Corinthians 13:4) by counting others more significant than themselves (Philippians 2:3), and even claim the honor of having the same mindset as Jesus himself (Philippians 2:5). The women in the Nkamira Transit Camp practiced listening skills. They choose to listen deeply to others and to God, becoming my trusted teachers.

LISTENING HEALS US PHYSICALLY

Empathetic listening can heal our bodies. The hippocampus is the seahorse-shaped part of the brain that controls the communication of memory, decision making, and warning signs. In cases of trauma, especially sexual trauma, the hippocampus can shrink by as much as 10 to 14 percent. Physical and emotional violence can affect a survivor's cognitive abilities long after the act is done, leaving a seemingly impossible road to recovery. Language centers go offline, leaving the survivor unable to answer the question, "What happened to you?" Decision making is impaired, leaving traumatized victims helpless to make informed choices at the moment they most need to. I wondered, *Are the women we now called our sisters doomed to a life of limited ability, but unlimited pain?*

When someone who experienced trauma shares her story with someone who genuinely listens, the brain actually regenerates itself. Much like a listening first-aid, over time, the hippocampus can be restored to its original size and health. Dr. Dan Allender, a Christian theologian and therapist focusing on biblical trauma recovery, says the hippocampus heals "through the process of reiterative, honoring storytelling and engagement. So, one just needs to stand back from that and say abuse is not only dark and evil, but the restorative process is simply God-honoring and beautiful." Dr. Brené Brown says, "If we share our story with someone who responds with empathy and understanding, shame can't survive."

> "*If we share our story with someone who responds with empathy and understanding, shame can't survive.*"
> BRENÉ BROWN

NOT SURE WHERE TO START?

Jesus raised the bar when he said, "A new command I give you: Love one another. As I have loved you, so you must love one another" (John 13:34). Much like the skill of perspective-taking, listening begins in one of two points of origin: self or others. When our listening begins from the point of self, we are forced to camp out in that region for the entire conversation. We aren't relating to someone else; we're only relating to our own experiences. Brave-soul listening invites others to grow, but self-focused listening reduces the humanity of the other. Empathetic listening embraces; self-focused listening excludes. As German theologian and activist Dietrich Bonhoeffer wrote, "Half-eared listening despises the brother and is only waiting for a chance to speak and thus get rid of the other person. Just as love to God begins with listening to his Word, so the beginning of love for the brethren is learning to listen to them."

For me, empathetic listening as a practice has been deeply convicting. I no longer blame "half-eared listening" on the mood I am in or on timing. Taking this conviction seriously was no small endeavor. Last year, I spent a season asking forgiveness for my self-focused listening over breakfasts, lunches, and dinners—sometimes from the same table in the same corner of the same restaurant for an entire day. Once, I remember ordering no less than six pour overs from a very patient server as I sat in a café for five hours, receiving three separate friends, asking forgiveness from each one of them. Two friends seemed to understand my listening regrets; one didn't. But all three forgave me. I've written emails and cards. I've made calls and sent texts. And I'm still calling, writing, and texting. I am still learning. But my regrets are turning into hope—and on good days, into virtue. I've found that people tend to want to forgive when they feel listened to.

What about you? Maybe you know you need to change, but do you know where you start? Maybe you feel like my son, Caleb. And you wonder, *How do I learn to listen?* Lessons are best learned when we take stock of who we are and how we behave. For example, I've taken scores of online, pen-and-paper, blog-post, and academic-study "listening tests." Some were so honest I had to take them twice, because I knew in my gut I wasn't ready to answer truthfully the first time. Yet each time I reflected honestly over my listening practices, I learned, even if at times it was only to recognize my limitations.

TIPS FOR LISTENING WITH EMPATHY

During the steepest parts of our climb, our guides walked alongside, offering us riddles whether we wanted them or not. They were checking to see if we were listening and still able to think clearly. Listening can be vital for your health and safety.

Empathetic listening requires practice and commitment, and its fruits are stunning. Remember, we are all designed to listen—and listen well. Any of us can begin with our very next conversation.

First, listen before you listen. Engage in *pre-listening*. If you're in a noisy location, ask yourself if you'll be able to hear the other person without interrupting or asking him to repeat himself. Can you focus? If not, move to a quieter place. This will speak volumes to the person you wish to hear. Because listening is often more a state of mind than a bodily circumstance, it's important to practice listening before you listen.

Stop for a moment. Where is your head? Your heart? Are they noisy? Can you honestly provide the speaker with your undivided attention? Stop multitasking. Give yourself generously to the moment. It's a sacrifice but worth it. Take a deep breath and quiet your thoughts. You need this to focus. If you allow silence after saying something, the other person is more likely to open up.

After listening, be quiet a moment. A small silence gives weight and allows reflection on both sides of the communication. Whether listening to a story in a war zone or a question from my sons, pre-listening has been one of the most powerful empathetic tools in my tool chest.

Consider the good Samaritan. In the parable, he came upon someone in an emergency, lying directly in front of him. Pre-listening would seem like the least reasonable thing to do. But listen he did. While others passed by quickly, he stopped. In stopping, Jesus allows his character to "hear" the story of a man who couldn't even communicate. He heard the situation well enough to find a solution amid the noise of cultural tensions, the threat of disease, the possibility of being attacked himself. He listened to the man's needs for compassion, healing, protection, and provision in a hostile land.

Second, we discover the person we think we know. Empathetic listening is all about listening to discover what the other person is trying to say—to discover who he really is, not who we think he is, to understand his pain, to isolate his problem, and even to midwife a solution. And more often than we may think, we discover something about ourselves in the process.

> By listening to and rephrasing what is being said, we use our imagination to, as the Japanese say, "Read the air."

Curiosity is the fuel of discovery. My friend Logan Wolfram, author of *Curious Faith*, often reminds me of this hope, "Belinda, we can give up our control for curiosity." Albert Einstein offered this directive to those who want to really live life: "Never lose a sense of holy curiosity." Curiosity is essential to empathetic listening, which requires us to rediscover both strangers and those we've known our whole lives.

Setting aside bias is key to cultivating the curiosity necessary to understand what is being said, not just what we want to hear (or not hear). By listening to and rephrasing what is being said (either out loud or mentally), we use our imagination to, as the Japanese say, "Read the air."

Facial expressions, emotions, circumstances, and power differentials all play a role in communication. For the Japanese, it's important to listen beyond the words, to be aware of all that surrounds the words, to read the very air that words float in.

In Jesus' parable, the Good Samaritan knew the infamous Jericho Road was fraught with blind turns and danger. The hero couldn't ask questions because the injured man was unconscious. So he read the air.

Now I realize my busy, tired, overwhelmed days, often infused with a touch of DKDC, could have been different if I had cared enough to read the air around me.

Third, be vulnerable. Listening with vulnerability requires humility—that is, not thinking more or less of yourself than you ought. Being vulnerable also means letting go of feelings of superiority or importance. It means letting down your defenses and letting go of the need to be correct and to react instead of consider.

It's easy to spot a conversation where vulnerability is missing. One person is busy prepping counterpoints rather than hearing what is said. Another is preoccupied with felt needs, while another is offering long-winded opinions on how to fix the problem. Vulnerability resists the urge to explain, defend, fix, or judge. It establishes mutuality; listening creates a context where someone can reciprocate, where trust has an opportunity to flow.

Years ago, Stephan and I attended one of Stephen Covey's 7 Habits of Highly Effective People seminars, back when it was *the thing*. I was eight months pregnant and dashing off to the bathroom often, so I don't remember much from the morning sessions. But I do remember one afternoon session. Maybe that's because it was after lunch (I was hungry *all* the time) or because I had slipped off my shoes and was comfortable again (my ankles were as big as an elephant's). I leaned in when the presenter opened the session with this habit: "Seek first to understand, then to be understood."

Listening to is one-dimensional and sympathetic, while listening into is mutual and filled with empathy.

People hunger for those who will listen *into*, allowing them to open the door to what is going on inside. Listening *to* is one-dimensional and sympathetic, while listening *into* is mutual and filled with empathy. Covey suggests we listen to understand what a person is trying to say in order to promote reciprocal listening. If this cycle is completed, trust and cooperation are built, leaving a tangible feeling of being respected and heard. To continue your exploration of listening, see appendix A to create your own personal listening inventory.

Each of us who climbed tasted the power of listening into our sisters in Congo. Of course, we were impacted by what they shared, but also by something else: how important our listening was to them. Our experiences were reciprocal. We were searching for their brave souls and hoping to find ours in the process. It seems, much like diamonds, souls have to be mined. And, along the way, we discover gems in ourselves too.

It is like the story of the Rabbi and his son, a young man training to be a diamond merchant. Living near each other, the two were in the habit of sitting and talking in the cool of the evening. As they sat, many neighbors and strangers alike would come to talk, to get advice, to *vetch*. Over the years, the son had patiently watched his father give rapt attention and honor to each person he spoke with on those evenings, from the simple to the scholar. "Father?" he asked one night, "Why do you show so much care about even the silliest question or problem people bring you? Surely, all these people can't be that important to you?"

Knowing his son was training under a master gem seller, the Rabbi asked to see the variety of diamonds he was currently studying. His son complied, although he was surprised. Bringing out his bag of samples, his father gazed at the array of diamonds for a moment, and raising one up he declared, "Ah! This must be the most valuable of the whole bunch. Am I correct?"

The son deeply admired his father, his wisdom and grace. So embarrassed, the son did not want to contradict him. Yet the Rabbi persisted: "Is it, or is it not?"

Finally, the son relented and said no, it was not the most valuable. "But how could this be? It looks so beautiful. So large and bright."

"Father, you see, the trained eye can appreciate the true value of a diamond," said the son. "It is very difficult for the unpracticed eye to discern the real worth of a diamond."

Sitting back in his chair, the Rabbi folded his hands and smiled at the person now coming up his walkway.

"My son," he said, "the same is true with souls."

6

PEACEMAKING

Love is the only force capable of
transforming an enemy into a friend.

MARTIN LUTHER KING JR.

I've lived or traveled in many of the world's hot zones, including Northern Ireland, Serbia, Rwanda, Congo, Sierra Leone, and the Middle East. But teaching middle school was actually my first "war zone." Why? In a word, tribalism.

James was a short, thin, dark-eyed child with an easy smile and quick temper. I had never encountered a little boy with such big mood swings. He could go from a sweet-natured giggle to a jaw-clenching glare in a matter of seconds. He rarely yelled, but he often made his opinion known to those around him through name-calling and pointing out flaws in those who disagreed with him. He had an uncanny knack of faultfinding and belittling. Some might call him cruel, but I would say James was just forming his tribe in a destructive way.

One day I felt the gentle one-finger tap of our class worrier, August, on my shoulder. I turned to face a pale, teary boy. "Mrs.

Bauman, something happened in the bathroom," August said. After drying his tears and giving an understanding hug, I listened to his account. His friend Evan had gone to the bathroom and was coming out of his stall when James confronted him. Evan loved anything that *lived*. He talked constantly of his pet birds, rabbits, chickens, goats, squirrels, spiders, and snakes. He often came to school without remembering his socks, but always remembering to put some small critter in his coat pocket. Most of the kids thought Evan was funny, but James thought he was a threat.

James had pushed Evan just hard enough to topple him into his own unflushed pool of urine. According to August, Evan had turned around and told James to "knock it off." Small as he was, James used his weight to slam Evan against the bathroom wall and began choking him. Then he threatened, "I'll make every day of your stupid life miserable as hell." When James finally let go and left, Evan slumped down to catch his breath while August sheepishly peered out of the adjacent stall and asked if he was okay.

My lesson in tribalism was still unfolding. Evan decided to speak up for himself and tell his parents of the bullying incident. Meanwhile, several of the boys in the class aligned with James, who had told his own version of the story to his parents. Each set of parents sought allies and used terms like "bully," "socially awkward," and "bad influence." They found sympathetic ears in other teachers, forcing the administration to consider whose side their board members were taking. Board members worried about what the school's biggest donors might think.

In the end, both boys mumbled, "I'm sorry." But neither sets of parents nor their allies could stomach being in the same room together. By the time seventh grade rolled around, only one boy, James, returned. Evan did not.

Tribalism had won; our school was split. James and Evan had watched as lines were drawn, sides were taken, and names were whispered—all strategies in how *not* to love your neighbor or your enemy.

The very human trait of seeking out those we "belong to" can be creative or destructive. Finding and standing with our tribe is a positive thing, but defining our tribe—who we are—by who we are *not*, by who we stand against, or by who our enemy is, tears our world apart at the seams.

Middle school marks the beginning of searching for beliefs and values, and for trying out behaviors to see if they suit us, asking the whole way, "Who the heck am I, really?" In essence, the search for a tribe is the search for identity. This is where a sixth-grade war zone mentality takes hold and where we learn to define ourselves by who we call our enemy.

Do not be deceived. The battle begins when we draw the line between our tribe and those we call traitors.

> *Do not be deceived. The battle begins when we draw the line between our tribe and those we call traitors.*

While a tribe mentality can begin to form in elementary school, in middle school it becomes the Holy Grail. It is only human to want to belong to an "in group," but this innocent desire can quickly lead to the creation of the enemy "out group." Those left in the middle must fly below the radar; they must remain undetected or risk having to choose a side.

Ten years after the episode with James and Evan, I'm still tender toward the adolescent angst that defines twelve-year-olds. When your deepest question in life is "Who the heck am I?" the road ahead is going to be long and filled with potholes. Evan was searching for his tribe, and James believed he was protecting his. Both boys saw the other as the problem, not as a person. Evan was definitely the victim of violence and bulling, but he responded to this violence by turning off his radar to James's humanity. James never recognized his insidious campaign to characterize Evan as someone who could never be part of his tribe, a dehumanization that slowly robbed Evan of his personhood. And, most terrifying of all, this cycle played out over and over again at all levels of the school, slowly eating up the humanity of everyone who engaged in the stereotyping and side-taking that ensued.

And so it is with all of history.

THE NEED TO TRIBE

Our need to be a member of a tribe is real, and finding our tribe can be tremendously liberating and energizing. The moments when people echo, "What! You too?" or "I thought I was the only one," are the moments when friendships are born. Our need to identify and align, to be known and accepted, is healthy.

What is *not healthy* is our perceived need to create an in-group and an out-group to form our identity. Whether that involves middle school bullying or sophisticated evangelical identity politics, any time we knowingly or unknowingly disengage perspective-taking and empathetic listening for the sake of tribe, we dehumanize the outgroup.

With his disciples, Jesus often addressed the fundamental human need to tribe, and he never gave an inch on what the "good tribe" should be. Tribe, according to Jesus, is one formed and moved by love—world-changing, wound-healing, mind-blowing love. For a glimpse into Jesus' view of tribalism at its best and at its worst, look no further than the Sermon on the Mount. For example, he said, "But to you who are listening, I say: Love your enemies, do good to those who hate you, bless those who curse you. If someone slaps you on one cheek, turn to them the other also" (Luke 6:27-29).

Jesus was saying something like this: tribe is great and, in fact, was my idea, but only under one condition, with one purpose above all others. Tribe is not the basis for sorting the sheep and goats. It is not permission to decide who's in and who's out. And it certainly isn't your excuse to bypass your heart or your brain. No, the singular purpose for tribe is to know and show love.

ONE PURPOSE ONLY

Our world today is full of terrifying headlines: violence in the streets of Syria, Congo, and Bethlehem. Protests over police brutality, political oppression, and military occupations. Terrorism in the form of vehicles plowing into crowds in Paris, Berlin, Stockholm, London, New York City, and Toronto. A sea of refugees flooding the banks of Greece, Jordan, and Lebanon while America turns most refugees away.

Yet these problems are not only far away. From mall and school shootings, domestic violence, and road rage to schoolyard bullying, sexual exploitation, and violence, our world is angry. Passive-aggressive behavior is epidemic, and sarcasm is now a full-blown American pastime. Given this, it's no surprise that sixty million Americans suffer from what sociologists call chronic loneliness. As we grow more disconnected, isolated, and distant from the human community, we grow less good, less true, and less beautiful—and more incapable of knowing even ourselves.

"When the enemy has no face, society will invent one," says journalist Susan Faludi. We turn the tribe into traitors. We imagine our enemy—they, them, those who are against us, whether across the world, across the aisle, or in the cubicle next door. We cave into the lesser angels of our nature, draw lines, and hide behind them. We drink in complacency as if it were medicine. Fear starts to swell. And when we become afraid, everything inside us wants to stop. We lose sight of our purpose and stop caring altogether.

Too much evil.

Too much suffering.

Too much to be afraid of.

When we stop caring, we stop loving. And when we stop loving, we stop doing. We trade messy for quaint, gutsy for tame, authentic for fallacious. We settle for less. We seek to be pampered. We rationalize sympathy, apathy, and even antipathy.

Nowhere else is the loss of purpose more apparent than in our stories of conflict. Yet every good storyteller will tell you that if there is no conflict, there is no story. Stories hinge on leaning into the tension of a conflict and believing, even if just for a moment, that it can be resolved. Isn't the word of our testimony actually our stories of attempting to overcome conflict on this side of heaven? Yet conflict will be ours to overcome as long as we are here on earth. Don't be fooled; the choices we make while in the midst of conflict determine how our story will end. In the very crucible of enmity, heroes are formed. And sometime the heroes are "sheroes."

Let me introduce you to Elsie.

WHAT IS RUNNING INSIDE YOU?

"There's an old proverb here in Rwanda," Elsie said over her cup as she talked. "You can outdistance what is running after you but not what is running inside you."

> *"You can outdistance what is running after you but not what is running inside you."*
> **RWANDAN PROVERB**

Both were key to her survival.

During one of our return visits to Rwanda, Elsie and her husband, Nicolas, and their children joined our family for lunch in Kigali. We hadn't seen each other for years, so returning to Rwanda was full of reunions and remembering. But something was unusual about this lunch. As we sipped African chai and let the children wander the gardens, she told me a part of her story I had never heard. Looking back, I know why she had finally shared it. I had asked her a question, and somehow, she could tell I intended to listen, to lean into the tension of her perspective.

"Elsie," I said as she put down her tea. "God is asking me to listen to the stories of women who survive the pain of war and to tell anyone who will listen about their reality and their bravery." Her brown eyes looked at me with kindness. She knew what was coming.

When the genocide tore across Rwanda in 1994, Elsie and Nicolas were newlyweds. Nicolas, being of the Hutu tribe, had to figure out how to protect his new Tutsi bride from the Interahamwe militia. The term "tribe" had taken a deadly turn, and "Hutu" and "Tutsi" became false and diabolical codes for "in" or "out." Because of this, Elsie spent many nights hiding—in ditches, in closets, under beds. Eventually Nicolas risked his life by forging Hutu identity papers for her, and together with their new baby, they escaped to Congo and found safety. With help from a Scottish friend, they were able to resettle temporarily in Scotland where Nicolas earned his PhD in applied entomology and their family grew.

Nine years post-genocide, Nicolas's hope for Rwanda was in farming together with war widows and adult orphans, the work aimed at holistically transforming lives of these local rural small farmers and their communities. He calls the business *Ikirezi*, which means "precious pearl" in Kinyarwanda.

While Nicolas and Stephan discussed community-interest agribusiness, Elsie stared at her tea, lost in a memory. My mind was percolating with questions: *After such evil, how could two tribes at war forgive one another? How could Elsie trust her nation enough to return? How do a husband and wife rebuild their family?*

In the end, I landed on a more important question: "Elsie, how did you heal?"

We ordered more tea, and Elsie began to unwrap the rest of her story like a fragile gift. She told me they didn't find out what happened to their families until they returned to Rwanda. Nicolas had lost his younger brother to extremists when he was unable to provide adequate identification. His brother-in-law was chased out of his home and torn apart by dogs used by the local militias, who were his neighbors, schoolmates, and members of his church youth group.

"We returned to a country devastated and struggling. Nicolas's father and mother were still alive, but so many we knew were lost," Elsie said as she looked out over the valley beyond the cafe. "But it was harder for me. I had lost everyone. Belinda, I had nothing to go back to except fear and deep, deep anger." Glancing away, she told me that when she looked into the eyes of her neighbors, she knew they were also the ones who had killed her family, taken her land, and looted her home. Her neighbors had become her enemies.

Elsie had been plagued by depression, thoughts of death, and nightmares. And so many questions—horrible questions. How could a man smash a baby's head against a wall? How could a woman lift a finger to point the way for a machete-wielding crowd, betraying the children her kids had recently played with? How could neighbors become traitors?

Elsie called this her "great darkness." Once in Scotland, when life became unbearable, women from her church anointed her with oil, laid hands on her, and prayed the word *resurrection* over her again and again until she felt it settle into her heart, a light against the darkness.

"How did I heal?" she mused as she gently rested her teacup in the palm of her hand. "How did I heal?" she asked again. "Belinda, the words 'I forgive you' have been my road to freedom."

> *"How did I heal? The words 'I forgive you'*
> *have been my road to freedom."*
> ELSIE

I thought I knew what forgiveness was: pardon, absolution. An exoneration granted after sufficient remorse was displayed by the offender. A forgive-and-forget arrangement. But Elsie and so many other women who have survived the violence and injustices of war, have taught me that forgiveness is more about the forgiver than the forgiven. It's much more about choices made, paths taken, and actions executed than moral-sounding pleas and platitudes. When real forgiveness is granted, it's steeped in the hard work of knowing the God who forgives and the one we are forgiving, even if that person is a court-certified traitor.

Elsie would eventually learn the horrific details of how her parents, siblings, aunties, uncles, and cousins all died at the hands of those she had once called neighbors and friends. Years after the genocide, the newly established government was overwhelmed with the amount of court cases concerning murder, rape, and torture that needed to go to trial. As people waited for justice, there were rumors that revenge would be taken if the hundreds of thousands of cases were not heard more quickly. Both defendants and plaintiffs were suffering and growing angrier by the day. By the year 2000, 130,000 people found guilty of genocide had been placed in Rwanda's burgeoning prison system. At that rate, it would take another hundred years to try all those cases. Elsie was one among many, so when she was offered the opportunity to engage the traditional Rwandan system of justice known as *gacaca*, she said yes.

I learned about gacaca by watching it. The outdoor court was held each week on our neighborhood street corner, and the boys and I took walks to observe. Gacaca means "justice on the grass." It's an old system, predating colonialism. Conflicts between Rwandans were traditionally solved by all those concerned sitting down on a patch of grass that was "soft enough for everyone," and where each party stated his or her case. For Elsie, and many like her, the gacaca courts became a trusted alternative to the belabored formal court system. The judges, jury, and decisions were all local, and as much as the perpetrator was known, so was the victim. Each was at one time considered a neighbor. Judges and juries could try everything from property damage to murder and impose sentences of up to life imprisonment, but not the death penalty. Under gacaca leadership, there were serious consequences for serious crimes.

The closer the day approached for Elsie's gacaca trial on behalf of her father, the more she wrestled with her choices. Once there, she came face to face with those who murdered her family, looted and pillaged their land. Elsie loved Jesus and knew his way. When she looked at their faces and heard their stories, she knew she did not want revenge. Yet she also knew she could not simply "forgive and forget." What did justice look like for her, her family, and her tribe? How could she heal? She described a crucial moment:

> In my weakness and exhaustion, I said, "Lord, I want to give you back my right of judgment and make you the judge, for my people, they are yours, and my life is yours. But I am tired with the things that I must understand, and since I can do nothing to help my family, I can see that I am losing the case!" And I clearly heard God say this: "Forgive them because they

did not know what they did. But Me, I know, and they are Mine too. I know them all, and I love them."

And I clearly heard God say this: "Forgive them because they did not know what they did. But Me, I know, and they are Mine too. I know them all, and I love them."
ELSIE

Then Elsie fell silent for a long time. The true cost of loving others as God loves them—friend and enemy—had been made clear. Could the grace of God really reach that far? Could empathy transform the neighbors who had killed her family from traitors into a more powerful kind of tribe?

Elsie began to plan her course of action. Gathering her courage, she crafted a letter to the gacaca judge who was trying her case and explained that she desired to forgive her neighbors formally for the crimes they had done both to her family and to her tribe. She asked the judge for only one thing: the right to meet with those involved and with their children once a month so she could help them understand human rights, crimes against humanity, the love of God, and his good plan for all.

On the day the judge fully granted her request, Elsie said her "great darkness" transformed into great light—not only for her as a survivor but also for the land soaked with blood and those who spilled it.

Our tea was now cold, and tears were streaming down my face. I had to hear more. Conflict transformed by empathy seemed so costly—so hard. "What happened?" I asked.

"More than you could ever imagine, Belinda," Elsie said. "Infinitely more than you could ever ask or imagine." The way of empathy transformed Elsie's monthly visits to her father's village into conversations about crops and cows like her family used to raise; into well-paying work for those living there; into a solid, well-built church the whole community saved funds for and worked on for two years. Elsie's choice to engage empathy transformed decades of ignorance and intolerance into a good, solid education in a new school building for every village child, no matter their family's tribe, trade, or transgressions.

Elsie's extraordinary act of empathy transformed an overwhelming conflict into a grace-soaked opportunity. And where antipathy and revenge could have taken root, today Elsie and her former enemies have forged a friendship, a new community, a tribe.

"So you can see why, try as I might, God would not let me outdistance what runs deep inside me," she said, eyes beaming with joy.

FROM COLLISION TO CHOICE TO CHANGE

But just because you can see the train coming doesn't mean the impact is any easier. When conflict arrives at our door and lives crash into each other, what is the role of empathy?

If conflict is neither good nor bad—just is, has been, and always will be—then could conflict be beneficial? Could we walk through our lives welcoming conflict as beautiful collisions, not rejecting it? It isn't how we feel about conflict but what we *do* with it that can yield positive change. The deep discomfort felt during conflict can't be varnished over with Hallmark-card sympathy. It refuses to be ignored through our attempts at sophisticated apathy, and it rebels when we intellectualize our weapons-grade antipathy.

What if there was a totally different path? And what if it was up to you?

Our choice to engage in or ignore the disciplines of empathy in the midst of conflict can result in creative change or a soul-sucking energy drain. When we choose the way of empathy, our life collisions can transform opposition into opportunity. Elsie proved this true in the worst of situations.

So why not us?

The way of empathy is less a freeway from point A to point B than a trail navigating the boulders on an ascending mountain path. It may not be easy, but it moves us forward. On a path with clear trail markers we can navigate by, difficulties can lead to choices, and choices can lead to change. We know good choices lead to creative solutions and positive change, and bad choices entrench contention and prevent change.

Though embracing conflict can create beauty, it will never be comfortable. Tension in our relational or cultural contexts affect all other areas of our lives, and many of us avoid conflict at all costs. For some, conflict is best when it blows up, like a bomb, as quickly as possible, diffusing the discomfort.

The fight-or-flight response to conflict originates in the part of the brain called the amygdala. This tadpole-shaped area is incapable of distinguishing between a real threat and a perceived one. So whenever you *feel* threatened, your amygdala is causing it. On occasion, the reaction is so intense it triggers a freeze response. We sometimes call this extreme version of fight or flight being "emotionally hijacked." Our collective amygdala insists that, for the protection of the human species, we will never have a comfortable relationship with conflict.

But, according to University of Notre Dame professor John Paul Lederach, known as a father of the peacebuilding movement, conflict is normal, no matter how uncomfortable it is. Yet we still want out. We ask questions like, "How do we stop this problem?" jumping directly from problem to solution, thereby bypassing any possibility of transforming the conflict. If we choose to press into the discomfort, we engage the root of conflict: our own hearts. Pressing in helps us to recognize we must pass through the empathy process, feeling the full weight of our collision, the choices we make toward those we collide with, and the change that is wrought. Our personal, relational, cultural, and even structural choices can humanize or dehumanize those we really want to punch (fight) or hide from (flight).

Lederach suggests that real conflict is never just an isolated incident, and therefore if we fight or flee once, we're very likely to do it again and again. On a microscale, this way of being in the world is likely to cause deep personal pain and alienation, and even self-sabotage. On a macroscale, this way of being in the world is how wars begin and become entrenched, whether internal like Rwanda's or external like the conflict between Israel and Palestine. Wars can simmer at a low boil for decades.

Conflict has a process structure of circular episodes connected together like a Slinky (remember those?). Because conflict episodes are circular, you run into the same responses to conflict every time—unless change happens. Circles have benefits though: they always come around to the same spot again and again, and if you map them as you go, they can provide indicators for which adaptive responses or empathy skills can transform conflicts into possibilities. Think of this as a "been there, done that" map. Just like a Slinky, conflict episodes can move in a linear direction, forward or back, providing clear progress over time. When conflict hits, this model becomes a "transformational platform," changing our fight/flight questions, such as, "How do we get rid of the problem so we can go back to the way we were?" to transformational questions like, "How do we change the way we do things so things like this don't happen as often, or hurt as much?"

A friend and longtime hero of mine, Duane Elmer, confronts conflict with a similar model. By entering our "cultural incidents," as he calls them, with our eyes open, we can recognize and make choices leading to increased understanding. If we don't, we risk entrenching stereotypes and growing bitter. These choices can make the difference between a restored or failed relationship, and a culture of war or a culture of peace. The stakes are high.

Both Lederach and Elmer suggest that the key to embracing conflict—and especially transforming conflict—lies in choices we make from the epicenter of our identity: our soul. Today any action you take, any decision you make, or any response you have to conflict will involve a soul either at war or at peace. Who we are at the core affects how we engage our choices. Do not be deceived. Choices provide the very platform for change—peaceful or destructive—and create around us a whole world of tribe or traitors.

Elsie found that no matter how hard she tried, she could not outrun what was inside her. The collisions she experienced were both culturally and relationally complex. Her choices were very personal. Her identity as a Tutsi Rwandan, as a woman, as a daughter, and as a wife were all confronted. Her discomfort was extreme, manifesting as post-traumatic stress disorder and depression. Her desires to fight and flee were also extreme. A government system that had once protected her had turned on her. Her neighbors had hunted her like an animal. Her childhood friends had killed her family and stolen her father's land.

Weighed down by sustained, complex trauma, Elsie's amygdala hijacked her ability to make decisions, at times causing her to freeze up for days. With help from compassionate people who listened carefully and leaned into the pain of her story, Elsie came back online. Nicolas worked hard to understand her perspective as a Tutsi wife of a Hutu man. Her Scottish friends prayed for her, anointing her with oil for healing and transformation. In fact, the empathy shown toward Elsie helped her practice empathy toward those she considered traitors, ultimately helping her make choices that affected hundreds of lives. What choices did she make?

- Choosing to not curse her husband's Hutu tribe, she blessed her own identity.

- Choosing to forsake revenge, she engaged the gacaca courts and stopped fighting.

- Choosing to return to her father's land to face those who killed her family, she stopped fleeing.

- Choosing to forgive them, she ensured they would not forget so it would never happen again.

- Choosing to be with them, to work with them, to learn with them, to build with them, to grow with them, and to worship with them, she transformed the fear and pain of death into a community of life.

For Elsie, there was nothing quite as stunning and beautiful as watching her father's land, stained red with blood, shake off the shadow of death and begin to bloom. She said, "Before the genocide, we used to say, 'Life is in the cow.'" By giving cows to her former enemies, Elsie chose to restore life not only to them but also to herself and her family. Change came when together they planted crops for health and flowers for beauty. Change came when together they built houses for protection and schools for prospering.

The deepest change came when they established a church so the One who transforms could take up residence there. By choosing to worship together in a land where many priests were complicit in genocidal ideology, where religious men and women had succumbed to violent tribalism, and where many churches had been places of slaughter, they transformed their very identity from traitors into tribe.

"The church knows something more," Elsie reflected. "Something beyond presidents, museums, and memorials. The church knows the deeper process, the ancient power of love."

BLESSED ARE THE PEACEMAKERS

Peacemaking is not linear. But as I said, it isn't completely circular either. It resides in the space between the spaces—the now and not yet, the I am and I will be. Our identity is always being transformed, so why would we expect our ability to resolve conflict—with its deep roots in our identity—not to occupy similarly fluid ground?

I love the way my Arab-Israeli-Christian friend Dina explains it. Her story, like Elsie's and Esperance's, is filled with many beautiful collisions and difficult choices, forming the bedrock of her ability to transform opposition into opportunity. As you can imagine, her world is filled with conflict. Her very identity is a challenge to everyone around her on some level. "Each time I introduce myself, I am aware of the many levels of identity I have," she says.

First, I am a Christian. I was born as a Christian. . . . I am also a Palestinian, culturally. Unfortunately, Palestinians are perceived as Muslims and terrorists. That is not correct. I assure you, I am not a terrorist. I have a heart full of God, like to serve Him. The third label of my identity, I am an Arab. In the mind of the Western being, an Arab is equal to being Muslim. That's incorrect as well. Not all Arabs are Muslims. Arab predates Islam. . . . And I am an Arab Palestinian. . . . The fourth label of my identity, I am an Israeli. I was born in Israel and I have Israeli citizenship. And I am a woman. You know, in the Middle East, women are the most disadvantaged sector of the community, because they are not only part of an ethno-political minority, but they are living in a patriarchal community.

So, what is Dina's secret to addressing conflict? It is her "death grip on the one purpose," she says. Jesus gave his disciples a command that they love their enemies (Matthew 5:44). According to Dina, any time we define ourselves by our tribe, we are bound to discover enemies. All tribes draw lines deciding who is in and who is out. All tribes disconnect from each other at the very moment they are connecting within themselves. For her, each level of identity is personal, and all of them can spark conflict. She suggests that each level is charged with myths—myths created by others, and myths created by ourselves. These myths fuel the values that form behaviors and ultimately legacies. She says, "Wherever there are tensions between me and someone else, that layer of my identity suffers. . . . I am not at peace with someone who challenges any part of my identity, except one: my identity as a peacemaker."

This final layer, the peacemaker, is not challenged by tension or tried by myth. In fact, wherever there is conflict, our identity as peacemakers rises to the challenge. "When there is conflict," Dina says, "this is the layer we must let rise to the top first. Using this perspective, we do not react to the tension; we respond from our hearts. We engage our identity because we know we are needed to transform the conflict."

Dina believes that engaging empathy with a heart of peace has transformed all areas of her identity. She represents hope for the Middle East and for us too.

MIGHTY BE OUR POWER

Holy empathy can transform despair into hope. And people who experience this kind of empathy are very likely to *act* empathetically.

Motivation to change what is troubling, painful, and even intractable begins to rise. Yet it's easy to get sucked into negativity when staring down the barrel of a loaded power struggle between tribes. No one knows this better than Nobel Peace Prize winner Leymah Gbowee. She grew up during the brutal Liberian civil war, married into a violent marriage, and after years of suffering, she began to disbelieve that God heard her cries for rescue. She almost gave up.

Why didn't she?

If you were to ask Leymah and her army of women-turned-world-changers what superpowers they used to transform one of the most protracted conflicts in the world, they would give you a very simple answer: they listened to one another. They labored to see through each other's eyes. And most of all, they prayed together. Leymah believes the idea of praying together came to her one night directly from God. She said, "I couldn't see a face, but I heard a voice, and it was talking to me—commanding me: 'Gather the women to pray for peace!'"

> *"I couldn't see a face, but I heard a voice,*
> *and it was talking to me—commanding me:*
> *'Gather the women to pray for peace!'"*
> **LEYMAH GBOWEE**

To "overcome evil with good" (Romans 12:21) in the midst of their conflict, thousands of women gathered in peace and protest as the Women of Liberia Mass Action for Peace. Each woman acknowledged her tribe: Muslim. Christian. Women. Girls. Together, they became a force bent on transforming the death of their children into education, food, and futures for all children.

Mighty be their power.

Their prayers and chants every day revolved around a simple request to a peaceful God, and to the violent men who held the power to turn their country from war into peace:

We want peace. No more war.
Our children are dying—we want peace.
We are tired of suffering—we want peace.
We are tired of running—we want peace.

PART THREE

NOW, TAKE
YOUR RISK

*And the day came when the risk to remain tight in a bud
was more painful than the risk it took to blossom.*

ANAÏS NIN

7

OBSTACLE ILLUSIONS

Strength doesn't come from what you can do.
It comes from overcoming the things
you once thought you couldn't.

RIKKI ROGERS

The phrase "it's all downhill from here" takes on an entirely new meaning when you're on top of Kilimanjaro. While planning our trek, one of our outfitters offhandedly quipped, "If you think the climb up is hard, just wait till you come down."

Abraham met us at the lodge the night before our climb. He handed out maps, advised us on how to stay healthy, how to walk, how to breathe, and how to get enough calories on the mountain. His counsel was based on decades of experience; he had summited Kilimanjaro more than two hundred times. His final advice of the night? "The descent will test you, Mama." His smile was kind yet serious. "But remember this: by climbing up, you are made stronger for coming down."

> *"By climbing up, you are made
> stronger for coming down."*
> ABRAHAM, LEAD KILIMANJARO GUIDE

Holy empathy has the power to save us. But the journey can be costly and the illusions daunting. Just like Kilimanjaro. By all physical accounts, we were exhausted as we descended. During one stretch, Alyce and I took ten steps then stopped to rest, then ten more steps before resting again. We were braver than when we had started. We had more grit. The mountains we had climbed—both Kilimanjaro and the mountains inside us—had given birth to new tenacity within us.

But was it enough?

Huge flakes covered Leia's eyelashes as she plopped down in front of me and leaned back on my knees to rest. I pulled her close to me for warmth as she shut her eyes. "Hey, Mama, you okay?" I whispered in her ear. She answered that she was fine. But the look in Ruth's and Kris's eyes told me she was not. She admitted, "Well, I guess I blacked out and threw up coming back from the summit, but I don't really remember anything."

Blackout. Vomiting. Loss of memory. This was not good. All were signs of cranial edema. Rapid swelling of the brain is a big problem on Kilimanjaro. One look at the expression on our team nurse's face told me all I needed to know. Leia was in bad shape.

One of our faithful guides, Mustafa, placed his bicep firmly under Leia's armpit and began moving quickly down the mountain. Concerned, Ruth, Laura, and Kim followed close behind. They were all making good progress until Leia started bleeding from her nose. Afterward, she remembered nothing but feeling like she was in water. "When I closed my eyes," she would tell us later, "someone would gently slap me awake."

Halfway down the summit path, a woman called out, "I am a doctor." Seeing Leia in distress while passing her on the descent, and knowing how altitude sickness works, Dr. Christina ran down the mountain with the team, mentally rummaging through the medical supplies she had thrown in her rucksack back at base camp—anti-nausea meds, anti-inflammatory steroids, and an IV; exactly what Leia needed. Within minutes of arriving, Dr. Christina's IV brought life back to Leia.

Several hours before, Christina had been a complete stranger. Now she was Leia's life-saving physician. Christina said she had remembered us from the summit, especially the praying and singing. She had asked me if she could give her thumbprint in solidarity with our cause. She didn't know then just how much she would end up giving us.

The phrase "it's all downhill from here" still makes me smile. So much emphasis had been placed on preparing for the summit we didn't realize the real challenge would be leaving the mountaintop.

EMPATHY'S "OBSTACLE" ILLUSIONS

Some years ago, while gazing at what appeared to be a gargantuan (and grumpy!) barracuda through the thick glass at the aquarium tanks in Chattanooga, my then six-year-old son, Caleb, shouted, "Look, it's an obstacle illusion!" He had correctly perceived that the size of the fish was distorted but hadn't intended to create a pun. In his mind, *optical* and *obstacle* were one in the same.

And maybe they are.

You've probably encountered some of the recent backlashes against empathy. Questions about empathy seem to emerge every few years, especially when people plead for more understanding in the wake of the latest racist remark, sexist attack, social media gaffe, or political breach. Paul Bloom, author of *Against Empathy*, argues that empathy "distorts our reasoning, makes us biased, tribal and even cruel. . . . The problems we face as a society and as individuals are rarely due to lack of empathy. Actually, they are often due to too much of it."

Does empathy make us feel too much pain, distorting our perception and actions? Can it plummet us into unhealthy emotional terrain and ultimately depression? Do we listen to those who say, "The biggest deficit that we have in our society and in the world right now is an empathy deficit"?

Or maybe all of this is just a barracuda-sized obstacle illusion?

We were about to find out that the obstacles on the mountain were no more real or sizable than the obstacles we would face at home. Our journey homeward was a blur. Debriefing, luggage, an African market, journaling, and packing consumed our final moments together. On the return flight, some slept, some read, some devoured movies (a few even watched the film *Everest*). We flitted back and forth to each other's seats. Landing in Amsterdam, where we would go our separate ways, was bittersweet. As I stood at the gate to say goodbye, I felt the weight of having shared something big, something beyond myself, something that changed each of us. We knew each other so well—like sisters—that little needed to be said or done beyond whispered blessings and lingering embraces.

Many of us were tempted to shut down after we returned home. The intensity of what we had seen, what we felt, what we now knew and cared about, left us—as Ruth would say—traumatized. Many of us found it hard to sleep. Some found it hard to wake up. We all felt detached from both the life we knew before the mountain and the life we had come home to. We didn't seem to fit in either place. The cumulative effect of Ben & Jerry's coupled with Netflix binge-watching was alarming. Some of us cried more than we had ever cried before.

When we had hiked our final few miles together, picking our way over river stones for the equivalent of a half marathon, we had time to think about what we had done—both our successes and our failures. "Everyone will have one or two really bad days," advised a wise friend who had summited a year before. "Make room for that in your expectations."

For me, the transition home was filled with reflecting on the lessons I'd learned, on the love I'd both felt and given, on the risks I'd taken, and on the sheer audacious power of empathy to disrupt my life with the promise of setting the world right again. If learning is an act of creation, then God was creating in me what I longed for most: a brave and empathetic soul.

But I quickly learned I had more mountains to climb. I had discovered that the best—and perhaps the only—way to overcome obstacles is to become a student of what I fear most.

> *I had discovered that the best—and perhaps the only—way to overcome obstacles is to become a student of what I fear most.*

"Pain is a good teacher," Stephan likes to say.

"Empathy makes brave students," I like to say back.

But overcoming obstacles to empathy isn't easy. Sometimes we don't feel another's pain, or we feel her pain too much. Or our own pain hinders us from feeling altogether. By default, most of us fight or flee when facing suffering, but we can build our capacity to overcome obstacles. We can become stronger before we face challenges. On the mountain, the ascent prepared us for the descent, and the descent prepared us for home.

Brave souls know the signs of what Brené Brown calls "empathy misses," those missed opportunities to lean into empathy. The mountain descent—my obstacle illusion—awakened me to these missed moments. Since then, I've been trying to learn the signs.

As a team, we often responded to groans and complaints with "I feel your pain." Yet "I don't feel your pain" and "I feel your pain too much" summarize the two most daunting obstacles to empathy. God has given us science and Scripture to overcome them both.

But what if feeling or not feeling other's pain isn't the problem? What if empathy as a response to pain is actually the problem? Before we understand these obstacles to empathy—too much or too little pain—we need to address Paul Bloom's critique of empathy as "a poor moral guide." Bloom, a Yale professor of psychology, suggests empathy "drives people to treat others' suffering as if it were their own," which "motivates action" to take away suffering. Not a bad thing, right? But he claims our empathy is biased, and our blind spots distort our moral judgments, preventing us from making good choices.

That's a bold critique. But his logic is fundamentally flawed. He assumes empathy is exclusively about caring, not about caring *and* knowing. In our paradigm, caring without knowing is tantamount to sympathy, a disconnector. It's simply not true empathy. When employed correctly as a skill, empathy both *cares* and *does* something. Feeling the pain of another also motivates us to know more, to understand, to consider what our best response should be.

According to research psychologist at the University of Illinois Dr. Denise Cummins and her husband Dr. Robert Cummins, professor of philosophy at UC Davis, "Empathy is . . . a motivation to get us thinking—but then reason and deliberation should take over and dominate the subsequent discussion, judgment, or policymaking." Unfortunately, Bloom relies on only one dimension of empathy, the affective aspect—or emotional empathy, as he calls it—without including the cognitive dimension, which he calls "morally neutral" and "useful":

> Cognitive empathy is a useful tool, then—a necessary one for anyone who wishes to be a good person—but it is morally neutral. I believe that the capacity for emotional empathy, described as "sympathy" by philosophers such as Adam Smith and David Hume, often simply known as "empathy" and defended by so many scholars, theologians, educators, and politicians, is actually morally corrosive.

When empathy is pursued as both emotional and thinking, caring and knowing, Bloom's argument falls apart. In the end, he is debating semantics, his argument nothing more than an obstacle illusion. Don't let the barracudas scare you.

I DON'T FEEL YOUR PAIN

It can happen to any of us: we find ourselves in the presence of pain, and we feel precisely *nothing*.

After several days of collecting and writing war stories from women in dangerous places, I become numb. I hear the stories, and unless I have someone to process with, I can lapse back into my old timid and apathetic soul. I find myself cold, passive-aggressive, or indifferent. If brave-soul empathy truly is an unlimited resource for healing the world (and us), what do we do when we don't feel the pain of the person we are engaging?

Sometimes we need to pay attention to ourselves first. Our own anxiety is bound to hinder our ability to give. Do you know when your own issues stop you from caring for others? I know I didn't until I met Dr. King—not MLK, but nonetheless a pretty helpful guy.

When we lived in Rwanda, Caleb, then five, was diagnosed with Obsessive Compulsive Disorder (OCD). Today many people with OCD can live completely normal lives as they bravely lean into their strength. However, for a five-year-old living in post-genocide Rwanda, a profound stress built up for Caleb, exacerbating his OCD. His behavior became severe.

Caleb's doctor, Dr. Robert King from Yale Child Study Center, calmed us, reminding us that studies—even back then—indicated over 30 percent of the American population showed a moderate level of OCD. He helped us understand that our son was not alone and would need to learn to manage his issues in various circumstances. He reminded us what a tenacious little boy Caleb was. He gave us what he called his "best advice ever": we could learn to help Caleb by asking a series of simple questions based on the widely known acronym HALT:

H. Are you hungry? Becoming physically hungry can cause distraction from deeper issues that need attention, whether personal or relational.

A. Are you angry? Anger is often associated with a perceived powerlessness. When you feel you are out of control, you are tempted to fight or flee. When you feel powerless, you lose your sense of agency and responsibility to care. While there are dimensions of anger that are healthy, letting anger control you or hurt others is not healthy.

L. Are you lonely? Are you isolating yourself or having difficulty reaching out to your community? Keeping connected to those who know and care about you is key to keeping your own empathy levels high.

T. Are you tired? Becoming too physically or emotionally depleted is dangerous. Proper amounts of sleep (a Bauman house favorite!), quiet rest, exercise, and Sabbath-like days and vacations are vital to increasing our capacity to empathize.

I am grateful for Dr. King's best advice ever, not only for Caleb, but for me! I use HALT like *Star Trek*'s health scanners. As I scan for solutions to anti-empathy triggers, I am less likely to make these triggers my excuse. HALT has saved me more than once in places where a meltdown would not be good. It helps me pay careful attention to myself so I can pay attention to others.

At its core, empathy is a tool for comprehending others; a way to "read" others to understand them. When the old indifference, coldness, and judgmentalism creep back in, I know it's important for me to ask myself this question: "Are you able to pay attention to that person?" Asking if I'm *able* is very different from asking if I'm *willing*.

Consider the following practical ways to increase your ability to pay attention to a person you're struggling to empathize with.

Become situationally aware. Start with an easy one. What is this person wearing? Eating? Saying? What would a person in their tragic, boring, or joyful situation normally be doing? What do you feel as you think about this person? Are you anxious or let down? Excited or distracted?

Become a reporter. Asking the questions a reporter may ask can increase your attention span, even with people or issues you find personally hard to connect with. Examples include: What happens when someone drowns? What effect does chronic malnutrition have on a child's IQ? Why are so many young, black men incarcerated today? What is a rape kit, and why is it needed? What physical damage can be done by a close-range bullet or by fifteen bullets? Why would a woman be willing to become a sex worker?

What are the issues transgender teens face while growing up? What is the effect of heroin on the mind after one hit? Why would a mother risk fleeing her home to cross a border without proper documents? How do people with chronic depression hide it? What happens to the human brain when looking at pornography?

Nothing should be off the table. If you can ask it, you can find at least the beginning of a credible answer. In gathering information, you demonstrate caring and begin the journey to knowing about someone you once had no connection to.

Fake it till you make it. Sometimes learning to fake empathy can help you experience the real thing. No kidding.

When we first began listening into women's stories, bearing witness to the pain they carried, we quickly realized that empathies move in certain directions. We were motivated to know and care for rape survivors. However, we hit a major empathy obstacle when considering the perpetrators of these crimes. The sheer violence of the acts was so horrendous that it was hard for us to view those who could do such a thing as human. Sexual assault with broken bottles, machetes, and gun barrels left females as young as babies and as old as grandmothers butchered, bleeding, and fighting for their lives. At times, husbands, fathers, brothers, and pastors who have the opportunity to protect and help heal these women choose not to help due to the stigma associated with rape. Even more distressing is the tendency of families and communities to blame the victim, withholding any form of compassion altogether.

For a while, I made the mistake of keeping this struggle to myself, vacillating between guilt and anger whenever someone asked me about who was helping "the men involved," meaning the perpetrators and abandoning family members. *The men*, I thought, *are utterly lost and cannot be helped. The culture of rape has ruined manhood.* My weak understanding contributed to the dehumanization not only of the men but also of all people in these complex conflict zones. Did I support the culture of rape and the violent acts that went on with impunity? Absolutely not. But peace is not a zero-sum game, and empathy is not just for the good and right. Holy empathy has been given to us for all.

> *Empathy is not just for the good and right.*
> *Holy empathy has been given to us for all.*

As I wrestled with the implications of offering empathy to per-petrators, I was helped by what's called *empathic dissent.* By not backing away from intellectual and emotional dissonance, it's pos-sible to humanize even those you least understand or most dis-agree with. Faking empathy has helped me do this. Odd as it sounds, I had to learn to fake concern for the perpetrators in Congo. As I asked humanizing questions about the culture that boys grow up in and about why a man would join a militia that promoted rape as a weapon of war, I began to see how Congo's male youth were also victims in many ways.

I didn't have to fake it for long. I learned that some militias force boys to watch their sisters or mothers as they are raped. Sons and brothers are sometimes forced to rape family members. Some boys are themselves victims of rape. As I listened, I began to understand the fight many men were making against this culture of impunity, often putting themselves in danger. Many told stories about good men who snapped under the pain and humiliation of a system that uses sexual assault to dehumanize.

I knew I had made progress when Chelsea, our brilliant climb photographer, posted a breathtaking image of a young Congolese boy sitting in the doorway to the room where we had listened to pastors speak to us about their hope for peace and reconciliation. The boy was beautiful, close to the age of my youngest. Though Chelsea wrestled too, she believed the photo represented God's will to rehabilitate and restore, heal and bless the men of Congo. I broke and began praying human prayers for men who were perpetrators, because so often, they were the first victims. Dietrich Bonhoeffer urged, "We must learn to regard people less in the light of what they do or omit to do, and more in the light of what they suffer."

I FEEL YOUR PAIN TOO MUCH

For all the times we feel cold or indifferent, sometimes we feel too much pain. We become overwhelmed. Flooded. We may even shut down. Remember the hijacked amygdala?

Grief is one of those times. Dealing with the grief of others is complicated, especially when trying to manage your own.

Brenda, Stephan's sister, was a vibrant, beautiful lawyer living in Okinawa, Japan, with her equally brilliant, handsome husband, Lawrence. They had just moved so Lawrence could take up a new post with the army. Together they were raising two toddlers, with a baby on the way. When Brenda was seven months pregnant, Stephan got a call while we were having family dinner at our favorite local dive. Across the table, I watched Stephan turn ashen. "Brenda is dead," Stephan's father had said quietly, still shocked by the news. She had collapsed as she was descending the stairs and had hit her head on a sharp, tile corner. Lawrence had found her an hour later, but it was too late. The autopsy later revealed a congenital heart defect. She had lost consciousness at the top of the stairs, and she never woke up.

We remember Brenda with equal amounts of joy and sadness, but our pain paled in comparison to that of Stephan's mom and dad. Burying a child with her own child is a kind of grief from which one never recovers.

Yet even in their suffering, Jim and Carolyn opened their lives to others. One night a few months after Brenda died, sitting around the Bauman dinner table with friends, someone asked, "What happened that night?" For the first time, I heard my mother-in-law tell the story from her perspective. She recounted the call, the shock and disbelief, the river of tears and pleading with God, the numbness at the funeral home, the military guard, the army paperwork.

When Carolyn began to tell her story, one of the guests abruptly stood up and said, "I am so sorry. It's just so sad. I can't listen anymore. Please excuse me." It wasn't that she didn't care; after all, her eyes were brimming with tears. She just wasn't able to share the pain.

What happens to you when you encounter suffering? Do you feel a heroic impulse to respond, or do you feel yourself exposed and vulnerable, maybe even threatened? My days in war zones are filled with these encounters. In Congo, every encounter demanded each of us make a choice to lean in or step away.

Sometimes, I wonder why it took a war zone for me to lean in.

One of our greatest challenges as a team came while visiting the GESOM Hospital in Goma. Calling it a hospital is a stretch. There were no gleaming white walls, no smells of antiseptic. But the talented doctors and nurses were willing to take on cases abandoned by other local clinics, cases of women raped so violently they leaked feces and urine constantly even after multiple surgeries. These women could not work and therefore could not feed their children. Many of their families had rejected them, leaving them without any way to pay for their care. They were often sick and in pain yet brave enough to attempt four, five, even six reconstructive procedures. This small, hidden hospital was only whispered about, known as the place where women go when other hospitals, or even their own families, had given up.

As we toured the section devoted to caring for sexual violence survivors, the doctors and nurses told us details that broke our hearts. So many brave women, so many painful stories. We wrestled with shutting down, walking away, giving up. But Ruth pressed in. A writer, speaker, and orphan and adoption advocate, Ruth was playing with a bright-eyed five-year-old girl lying on her mom's bed. Her mother had survived multiple rape attacks and was having her fourth surgery in hopes of repairing her body and life. Ruth's voice trembled when, after the second playful fist bump the child gave her, she noticed an IV port in her tiny hand. Her mother looked away as she said, "Her surgery will be soon." This child of five was also a rape survivor. The pain of this realization drove many of us out of the room to catch our breath, stop our tears, and find our voices. As Ruth let the truth of the moment wash over her, she continued to play, composing herself and praying for them in real time. How did she do it?

Ruth asked herself how those two brave souls would want to be thought of: as victims or survivors? How would the girl on the bed feel if we couldn't stay? That day, we wanted to show this mother and baby girl they were heard, understood, and loved; that in their pain, they were ours—and we were theirs.

World Relief's Sexual and Gender-Based Violence program director, Dr. Esperance Ngondo, had recommended we give a gift of top-shelf Congo fabric to the women along with our attention and admiration. She said that by giving them the best, we were reminding them they were beautiful and deserved to be surrounded by beauty. As we handed the richly colored fabric to the women, we embraced each other as sisters embracing both joy and pain—especially our baby sister.

When we look at empathy strictly from our own perspective, sometimes we're limited by our ability to tolerate the pain involved.

"If you register empathy as a feeling that *happens* to you then, yes, there is a limit," says Dr. Emillana Simon-Thomas, science director for the Greater Good Science Center at UC Berkeley. "You have to numb yourself, or turn it into anger or hostility."

If empathy is something that just hits me blindside—for example, if my friend is dealing with depression, my son is failing in school, or my coworker just received a cancer diagnosis—I may feel resentful. Not long ago, I remember thinking, *I cannot possibly care about this right now. My friends and family need me, and if I give energy to this, I won't have enough for them.*

But remember what my friend Larissa said to me when she sent the image of Esperance's thumbprint:

> It's hard not to make it about me—oh, I'm so overwhelmed, I'm so tempted to ignore all this—the pain I feel for them. My pain.
> No.
> Their pain. Their rape. Their story. Their thumbprints. Their names. I can't do a disservice to them by saying, "It's too hard for me to bear." Those words in themselves are laughable.

If we define empathy from the perspective of the person suffering or from God's perspective, we tap into a sacred and unlimited resource. "Find a way to connect with it [the pain or joy], and, in that moment, you have an awareness you're not the person suffering," explains Simon-Thomas. "You can realize that your body is aroused and ready to act. If we can use that feeling as our Superman fuel to be able to support others, then there really is a never-ending supply of compassion."

When empathy is received as an invitation from God—an invitation that carries with it thick grace, the kind that surprises you with its strength—we connect with others in ways we may have considered impossible. As the apostle Peter wrote, "Be of one mind.

Sympathize with each other. Love each other as brothers and sisters. Be tenderhearted, and keep a humble attitude" (1 Peter 3:8 NLT). Love becomes distinctly tangible at that moment. Our minds, bodies, and souls become brave. Our love becomes real and our joy accessible, even in the midst of suffering.

God's command to make our love real, to empathize tenderly and tangibly with each other, does not hinge on our love being accepted or even noticed. We aren't promised applause, praise, or thanks. Through empathy, God asks us to give ourselves away to a vulnerable and angry world for the common good of all. That's not easy.

> *Through empathy, God asks us to give ourselves away to a vulnerable and angry world for the common good of all. That's not easy.*

We talk about vulnerability, authenticity, even risk, but we still fall short of action. Our willingness to move beyond the talk, to take a risk, to become vulnerable by taking up the mandate of empathy can set us free to become the kind of people we dream about.

EMPATHY FATIGUE

Empathy fatigue is real. The body of literature on it is expanding every day. Most is based on the cases of medical professionals, law enforcement officers, and first responders who daily confront physical and psychological suffering. Yet empathy fatigue can rise up in any of us, whatever our profession, location, or circumstance. People programmed to care can experience what neuropsychologists and trauma specialists call *compassion fatigue*, defined as "an extreme state of tension or preoccupation with . . . suffering . . . [which] can create a secondary traumatic stress for the helper." We see the faces of those ravaged by natural disasters. We hear the voices of millions on the refugee trail. We encounter stories about untold numbers of girls trafficked. The sea of suffering humanity overwhelms. It hurts too much, and we feel helpless. We shut down.

Even when we seek to help, pain is pain and joy is joy. Following God into the life of another person through the gift of empathy can be exhausting if we don't learn to modulate the pain we allow ourselves to feel. If we turn down the pain or joy we feel with other people too often, we run the risk of oversimplifying our understanding of them and their circumstances. If we keep their pain in front of us, we may lapse out of seeking to understand and simply seek to stop the problem.

So, what can be done to help those of us who feel overwhelmed?

Increase your soul awareness. Conduct a quick soul-scan by checking your HALT levels. Human beings are designed for balance, and whenever we become too hungry (physically or emotionally), too angry, too lonely, or too tired, we can face an empathy roadblock. Overcoming begins by simply caring for ourselves.

Respond, don't react. I've heard empathy described as the Wi-Fi that connects us to the situations and feelings of people around us. Neuropsychologists believe mirror neurons evolved primarily to help us deal with the folks standing in front of us. This makes sense in light of survival. Mirror neurons fire best when we are face to face with individuals who affect our daily outcomes. Reacting to the joy or suffering of someone immediately in front of us is an evoked form of empathy. Many researchers believe our sophisticated cognitive ability to perspective-take and listen empathetically evolved in humans relatively recently, thus requiring less recoil and a more reflective response. An overwhelmed reaction to tragic headlines is an example of reaction, not response.

The truth is, empathy is not a passive process. Simply reacting to someone in distress right in front of me is good, but if all I do is react to my biology—neuro-signals and action hormones—my soul is not engaged. It is God's design for humans to foster connection with both those present and those far away. It is also God's design for us to care for both those we naturally connect with and those we consider enemies. And it is God's design for those of faith to humanize all people, both friends and enemies, helping the world do the same. University of Michigan professor Dr. Stephanie Preston observed, "Only if you feel or actively foster a sense of agape (the Greek word for 'brotherly love'. . .) will you naturally come to feel a deep, emotional sense of empathy for people who are not part of your own social network." When in the midst of strong feelings, we don't have to react immediately; we can take time to reflect and respond.

Our mandate is to love everyone always. We are left without excuse.

Our mandate is to love everyone always. We are left without excuse.

Lean into soul-efficacy. Brave souls know this is hard work. They choose to be generous with their time, attention, and emotions. They choose to know and care. They choose to act.

Believing we are able to engage meaningfully and impact others through empathy relates to *self-efficacy*, or the ability to succeed in a particular task as determined by your mindset. Self-efficacy is the moment you say to yourself, "I got this."

We can apply this same concept to our souls. The capacity to connect deeply with others through empathy—let's call it *soul-efficacy*—is a dimension we often overlook. Soul-efficacy helps us to connect with challenging people. With soul-efficacy we can successfully connect with others at a core level, a soul level (thoughts, feelings, and actions). Soul-efficacy is based on God's design: healthy, holy empathy as an unlimited resource for those who are willing to learn and grow.

As a repenting and recovering high-functioning apathetic, I needed to know my primary obstacles to empathy. When rookie mountain climbers become a little too confident, experienced climbers are quick to remind them to "respect the mountain." Respecting the mountain means knowing the signs when it throws obstacles your way. When we know the signs, we respect the nature of the risk we take. Leia's was a life-or-death lesson, and she marveled at those who knew what to look for.

For each climber, Kilimanjaro created a certain amount of paradox, leaving us feeling, at times, a disorienting ambivalence. Joy and pain. Belief and doubt. Pride and shame. Respect and fear. Yet these emotions alone were never enough to lead us home. The grit we needed for climbing and descending was not found in *feeling* our way. It was found buried deep within our souls. A bravery of mind and heart so powerful, a motivation of will so audacious, that even the most breathtaking of obstacles became illusions before the God who saves us . . .

And you too.

8

EMPATHY AS A SPIRITUAL DISCIPLINE

You have watched my descent.
Now watch my rising.

RUMI

After years of living and working in Africa, I reluctantly took a trip to the Middle East. I was cautious because impossibilities seemed rampant there. That's why people say, "I'll believe it when there's peace in the Middle East." From history books to the evening news, optimistic views are hard to find. After tackling Congo, Kilimanjaro, and the mountain inside me, I felt the Middle East wasn't meant for me.

But something small kept niggling in the back of my brain: my birthright. I own my Jewish blood. Just ask my kids how often I can be found saying things like "He's got chutzpah!" Or, "Kind of shmaltzy, isn't it?" Or, if I am really pressed, a whirling of the finger at the temple and the cry of "*Mashugana!*" will suffice. Again with the Yiddish words! Oy vey . . .

Remember Grandpa Alexander? He hid his Jewishness most of his life—and from most of his family too. In fact, no one in my family had ever visited Israel, nor expressed any desire to do so. So when Lynne and our good friend Todd Deatherage invited me to travel with the Telos group to the land of my forefathers, I surprised myself by saying yes. What I found there was so extraordinary, I have returned every year since.

The Middle East—Israel, Palestine, Lebanon, Syria, Iraq, Iran, and beyond—fulfills its evening news stereotypes. Christians are both targets and instigators of religious persecution. Tension between Jews and Arabs is rampant, matched only by the tension between Muslim Sunnis and Shiites. Violence in Israel and Palestine is featured nearly daily in the press. Iraq seems to be a football passed between Russian, Iranian, and American hegemonies. And just as the Lebanese began to heal after thirty years of occupation by Syria, now Syrian refugees are flooding their country.

And the story of tribe and traitors goes on. Or does it?

If you dig a little deeper, you find something amazing. Deep empathy, the birth pangs of peace, is present in the Middle East. A few Israeli and Palestinian parents are sending their kids to mixed Jewish-Arab schools. One parent said, "We found a home here in our shared life, where we create something together that does not erase where we come from but builds a space with enough room for us all."

In another part of Israel, young kids participate in reconciliation groups as part of weekly playdates, so they can "learn to love 'the other,'" said one Arab mother. One organization, Musalaha (which means "reconciliation" in Arabic) is led by an executive board of Palestinian and Israeli community and church leaders. It hosts desert trips, summer camps, reconciliation training, and spiritual formation workshops as it works to humanize the enemy, fostering empathy through friendships. Others are leading efforts like the I AM PEACE campaign.

For some in the Middle East, empathy is deeply personal. Tala Jean, a tenth-grade student enrolled in the Peace Heroes curriculum at the Jerusalem School, changed her legal name because she was inspired by the Palestinian poet and spoken-word artist Mahmoud Darwish. Darwish champions the idea that small changes can make a large impact. Tala Jean, whose name means *candle*, said she wishes to be known as a candle in the dark in a land plagued by division. Changing her name was a small price to pay for something she hopes will have a big impact.

As I encountered these examples of empathy, something stood out in such bold contrast, I'm embarrassed I hadn't appreciated it sooner. Because empathy in the Middle East is so hard won and because large doses of courage and perseverance are needed to press on until there is fruit, empathy is fought for like a discipline. The people I met kept regular empathy rhythms—repeated, intentional, and deliberate approaches, methods, and programs that harness bold ideas. Many had curricula, some so well done they've been exported to other global hot spots. These disciplines are intended to confront the heart and head, dispel inhibiting emotions, and demand commitments to action that at times seem Herculean. Yet there is one simple goal: to make empathy accessible, practical, doable, and sometimes even fun—but most of all, possible.

If the spiritual discipline of empathy can change lives in the Middle East, it can change lives anywhere.

EMPATHY AS A SPIRITUAL DISCIPLINE

Dallas Willard defined spiritual disciplines as "activities undertaken to make us capable of receiving more of [God's] life and power." In other words, we pursue a spiritual discipline that is "an activity in our power that we do to enable us to do what we cannot do."

Quoting James S. Stewart, Willard says the heart of the gospel is "the continuous appropriation of the 'real presence' of Christ himself within the experiential life of the believer."

"I have been crucified with Christ and I no longer live," wrote the apostle Paul, "but Christ lives in me. The life I now live in the body, I live by faith in the Son of God, who loved me and gave himself for me" (Galatians 2:20).

Could it be we are called to display—like billboards in urban alleyways and on remote country roads—the awesome, severe, holy empathy of God? Is it possible to imagine God's empathy on display through our day-to-day courage, our conversations, our awkward attempts at compassion, our risks with perspective-taking, our best tries at listening, and our weak-willed commitment to embrace and transform conflict?

Many of us would probably respond, "Sounds nice, but it's absolutely impossible." To which God and the angels say, "Precisely!" Jesus said, "Apart from me you can do nothing" (John 15:5). So, yes, empathy is impossible. We may be hardwired for it, but engaging empathy is our choice. If we don't, we default to sympathy, apathy, or antipathy *every time*. Empathy is a spiritual discipline we pursue within our power so we can do something beyond our power. Something extraordinary. Something impossible.

Empathy is a spiritual discipline we pursue within our power so we can do something beyond our power. Something extraordinary. Something impossible.

That sounds like a superhero leaping tall buildings in a single bound, holding back speeding trains, or deflecting bullets with her hands. Even though superpowers sell movies, it's the invisible powers I'm after. The ones not as obvious.

Practicing spiritual disciplines can make us more loving, compassionate, and empathetic. Yet, Trappist monk and activist Thomas Merton wrote, "He [or she] who attempts to act and do things for others or for the world without deepening his [or her] own self-understanding, freedom, integrity and capacity to love will not have anything to give others." Practicing the disciplines doesn't automatically make us more empathetic. And certain disciplines just aren't practical for some of us—too spiritual, too removed, too disembodied from the dusty world in which we live.

Maybe they lack the heavy-lifting skills we talked about in chapters four, five, and six. With any spiritual practice, we run the risk of pursuing abstract concepts without *embodying* them in real life. Spiritual formation can become just a lofty exercise—an ideal one, an esoteric one, or even a rhetorical one.

C. S. Lewis illustrated this in one of my favorite books, *The Screwtape Letters*. Screwtape, a lead demon, advises his trainee to tempt his Christian subject when interacting with his mother, saying,

> Make sure that [the prayers] are always very "spiritual," that he is always concerned with the state of her soul and never with her rheumatism. . . . Since his ideas about her soul will be very crude and often erroneous, he will, in some degree, be praying for an imaginary person, and it will be your task to make that imaginary person daily less and less like the real mother—the sharp-tongued old lady at the breakfast table. . . . And, of course, never let him suspect that he has tones and looks which similarly annoy her. As he cannot see or hear himself, this is easily managed.

When we disembody spirituality, we pursue ideas about faith rather than faith itself. We become aloof, elitist, or even self-absorbed.

We sophisticate our apathy. We are religious without knowing it. Richard Foster wrote,

> We must not be led to believe that the Disciplines are only for spiritual giants and hence beyond our reach, or only for contemplatives who devote all their time to prayer and meditation. Far from it. God intends the Disciplines of the spiritual life to be for ordinary human beings: people who have jobs, who care for children, who harvest cassava, drive trucks, wash dishes, mow lawns, fetch water. In fact, the Disciplines are best exercised in the midst of our relationships with our husband or wife, our brothers and sisters, our friends and neighbors.

We have a brilliant friend, Mike Metzger of the Clapham Institute, who speaks eloquently of the theological concept called the "scandal of particularity"—the way in which God always expresses himself in *particulars*, generally through *people*: Mary and Joseph, for example, and Jesus himself, a carpenter's son from Nazareth. The Gospel stories include this adulterous woman, that Roman centurion, this tax collector, and so on. Love is always expressed, in Mike's words, as "this and that."

Empathy is impossible unless we pursue it like a spiritual discipline—in and through our daily lives, with people, for people, by people—not as a virtue or skill but as a daily rhythm where reflection and action are seamlessly stitched together, where grace and diligence meet each other every day through our successes and failures, breakthroughs and breakdowns. When we pursue empathy this way, we avail ourselves to oceans of grace we've never dreamed of, grace that can help us love in ways we never imagined possible—as "this and that."

SIX WAYS TO PRACTICE EVERYDAY EMPATHY

So where do we start?

In the year after our journey up Kilimanjaro, one question emerged again and again: What do we do now?

I wish I had known then what I know now. Although we jumped back into collecting thumbprints, speaking, writing, fundraising, and advocating, many of us found the old depressions, apathies, and paralyses were stalking us anyway. Mountaintop experiences can leave us depleted and even bored when we return to the valley. In the descent after the descent we learn to take on the hard work of everyday empathy.

For me, climbing Kilimanjaro was a quest, not an adventure. The difference? An adventure happens to you. You happen to a quest. A quest requires a question, a conflict, a mission, and a goal. Kilimanjaro was a grand quest to see if we ordinary humans could take on the extraordinary discipline of empathy to overcome an obstacle found both outside and inside us.

My quest? To love others as God loves them. Among the strongest lessons Esperance, Kilimanjaro, and my climb sisters taught me was about grit. Brave souls are gritty; they know that if they don't use it, they lose it.

Empathy is a discipline, so what we learn, we have to practice. Every day. No excuses—all the principles of spiritual formation apply. As Foster wrote, "Willpower will never succeed in dealing with the deeply ingrained habits of sin." Quoting Emmet Fox, he added, "As soon as you resist mentally any undesirable or unwanted circumstance, you thereby endow it with more power—power which it will use against you, and you will have depleted your own resources to that exact extent."

Holy empathy is impossible without God, and pursuing it as a spiritual discipline requires rejecting the *worship of our will* instead availing ourselves to the grace of God. Only then can we experience the audacious power of empathy.

But all this takes practice—and not the kind of practice that's divorced from the messiness of life. Below are my six favorite ways to incorporate empathy into everyday life. Some come from experts that know much more than I do. Some come by way of my climb sisters. Each puts into practice the empathy lessons we've encountered: perspective-taking, empathetic listening, and peace-making. All are possible to do now, as we are, whether we've climbed our mountains or are still anticipating the climb. But be warned: these activities are best carried out with a sense of humor, humility, and hope. They are risky, but that's the point. Brave souls become brave when we take risks—not just once but every day.

1. Engage art. Art can involve endeavoring to understand the human condition by exploring the perspectives and potentials of others. How? When we view art, we place ourselves in the mind of the artist. What was the artist thinking, feeling, and trying to say? In fact, the word *empathy* was developed as an art term involving what the viewer is feeling and what the artist intended him to feel when looking at a work of art. Art opens our souls to flourishing, and spiritual disciplines keep them open for creative solutions in the midst of beautiful collisions.

Whether you consider yourself an artist or not, always make time in your day for art. Buy a sketchbook and pencils for daily doodling. Look at your favorite new website's photos of the day, or spend time at the website of the National Gallery of Art or the Musée d'Orsay. Listen to a book or to music you wouldn't usually choose. I recently listened to Yale Law School graduate and Appalachian hill person J. D. Vance read his *New York Times* bestseller *Hillbilly Elegy* while I downloaded an old Johnny Cash album. Both were a reach for me, but both expanded my soul. I had the thought, *Wow, this is like the way I grew up,* about twenty times while reading the book, even though I'm from rural Wisconsin. And Cash's crooning brought these lessons home to my heart. Choose to listen, read, watch, and buy from authors, artists, poets, and musicians that are not of your color, culture, gender, or comfort level. This is what the word *empathy* was created for!

2. Shape shift. Whenever I'm in a line, I resist the urge to pull out my phone until I have shape shifted with at least one other person in line. Throughout time, folklore often featured mysterious beings "with the ability to become anyone or anything." Shape shifting is using your imagination to trade places with someone very different from yourself. To do this, pretend you've shifted your own shape to become theirs and then, in your mind, walk around in their lives for a bit. See what they see. Do what they do. What would they say? Eat? Love or hate?

I did this once on Kilimanjaro with our talented guide Lucy. I watched her walking and talking with Laura. Lucy was bright and animated, smiling and confident, and she wore fewer clothes than the other guides. She never used a walking stick, and she favored her left leg when hiking. As I considered her and the life experiences that I imagined made her so outgoing and confident, I tried to visualize her life off the mountain. I shifted into Lucy's shape. And because I still had five hours of climbing left, I carried it even further. I thought, *Now that I'm Lucy, what would she notice and wonder about me?* I tried to see myself through her eyes.

Curbing the temptation to laugh out loud while shape shifting can be a problem. It's also important to resist reducing the person you're shifting into. When you feel yourself begin to see through someone else's eyes, you may feel your empathy muscles building up, stretching your imagination and your emotions into unfamiliar territory. This is when you know you're getting a serious empathy workout.

As we spoke, wrote, and blogged, each member of our climb team retold the stories of women they'd met. Not only did they bear witness, but many of them also chose to feel the pain and joy so they could give voice to the perspective of our sisters, not just their own.

3. Say the magic words. While *abracadabra* may get you a rabbit out of a hat, it will not calm down an angry coworker or a sad child. Empathy has its own kind of magic called validation. In a world hell-bent on competing, many of us learn quickly that showing emotion or vulnerability can be equated with weakness. How often have you felt shame when showing emotion?

Expressing strong feelings about anything can also make the people around you feel uncomfortable. Discomfort can lead to others trying to put a stop to your feelings as soon as possible through reassurance, redirection, or even scolding. After years of learning it is *not okay* to feel bad, many of us wonder deep down if it's okay to feel anything at all. "Am I okay?" is a question everyone asks.

When our identity is challenged, we are likely to respond with defensiveness, anger, withdrawal, or even a little DKDC. Using words that validate someone's human experience communicates unconditional love and acceptance that can lead to healing in even the most complicated circumstances. Validating words take the heat out of the burn.

Validating words take the heat out of the burn.

Strong feelings, such as depression or anger, are real. They light up the same areas of the brain as physical pain. Feeling the same way as someone makes validation easy, and it's always important to validate honestly. Feelings are feelings—not right or wrong.

They just are. No matter how layered or complex, they are best communicated and validated first. Only then they can be addressed. Here are some magic phrases when talking with some expressing strong feelings:

- That makes sense.
- You are not crazy [or bad, or wrong] for feeling that way.
- I understand why you feel [name the emotion].

Increasing your empathy vocabulary to include words of validation is an excellent practice. A good place to start is with you. Next time you begin to shame yourself for "feeling too much," for example, try to say out loud, "You are *not* crazy for feeling this way." Empathy toward yourself is key to growing in empathy toward others.

4. Call a friend. The miracle of daily communication with friends worldwide has changed my life. On any given day, my husband or I can have conversations via email, text, Skype, Messenger, Zoom, and phone with coworkers, friends, and family on two or three different continents. I remember a day when this was unheard of. But now, in one day I emailed back and forth with a person in Congo, chatted with a friend in Lebanon, did a podcast interview with someone in North Carolina, and texted with a friend in England. One of the easiest ways to challenge yourself to grow in listening, perspective-taking, and acting on your empathy is to call a friend every day. It can be a wonderful way to learn empathy.

After arriving home from Africa, the team quickly devised a number of ways we could check in with each other. We Facebook, Zoom, email, and text. Sending images is key. I try to reach out to one of my climb sisters every month or so to ask one simple question, "How are you?" Then I open myself up for whatever comes next, practicing empathetic listening by listening to understand, not to fix, protect, or please—just to understand.

5. *Reverse engineer*. Sociologist Dr. Martha Beck suggests employing a technique akin to the process of reverse engineering to practice empathy. She advises working backward from the effects of an emotion to the emotion itself to reconstruct a better, more streamline and effective way to understand another person.

Start with someone who is a mystery to you, like your garrulous coworker, your introverted classmate, or your distant mother-in-law. "Remember a recent interaction you had with this person—especially one that left you baffled as to how they were really feeling," Beck proposes. "Now imitate, as closely as you can, the physical posture, facial expression, exact words, and vocal inflection they used during that encounter. Notice what emotions arise within you." What arises in you will be very close to what was going on in the person you seek to understand.

Recently I reverse engineered a man I was experiencing as bombastic and interruptive. I was speaking at a conference on women at risk, and after the talk, he approached me and said, "So, are you saying that men are the problem? That men are at the root of all the pain women experience?"

Uh oh, I thought. I was in the middle of writing this book and feeling very responsible for my empathetic vibes. I was at risk of disliking him a great deal, but I found that when I reverse engineered his behavior, I felt his fear and insecurity instead of anger. Like an animal feeling threatened, he made himself larger in the room so that no one would mess with him. My heart began to soften, and instead of dislike, I felt compassion. This led me to encourage him instead of fight him—or worse, write him off. I began by looking at him calmly and trying to smile warmly. "No sir, quite the opposite. I believe men are key to the solution!" Immediately he calmed down, and we went on to talk about what he, as a strong and capable man, could do to help protect women in war zones.

His thumbprint on our banner is one of my favorites.

6. *Make yourself uncomfortable.* Expanding your circle of empathy beyond people you naturally gravitate to is good for you. But like many things that are good for us, this practice is not always comfortable. When you take a seat on a bus, is there a type of person you aren't likely to sit next to? What about the homeless person you pass by every day on the way to work? Or the new coworker who could not be more different from you?

Highly empathetic people "do far more than empathize with the usual suspects," says empathy adviser and social philosopher Roman Krznaric. "We also need to empathize with people whose beliefs and values we don't share." What does this look like in practice?

Choosing to make yourself uncomfortable takes intentionality; it doesn't need to be complicated. Find a person you don't naturally empathize with and spend a moment with her. As you do, be aware of more than her words; become her student. Listen with your ears but also with your eyes. Your goal is to find one or two things you have in common with this person.

Are you uncomfortable around people of a certain race or sexual preference? Find someone and spend time getting comfortable. You may not understand the person fully, but knowing that you share a love for birds or burritos or the Packers or Trader Joe's is a good place to start. Make yourself uncomfortable by going to a gathering you wouldn't normally attend. Die-hard Democrat? Time to head to a Republican gathering. Evangelical Christian? Cross the street to visit the "everyone is welcome here" Episcopal Church. Stuck in a homogeneous reading rut? Engage and advocate for the writing, speaking, and perspective of someone not of your culture, race, or gender. Is your usual coffee shop in the east end of town? Time to cross the tracks and get a cup of joe on the other side.

The open and nonjudgmental side of empathy is often misunderstood. Some people believe that in seeking to understand someone else, we legitimize what we disagree with. No matter another person's politics, religion, or moral viewpoint, empathy doesn't reduce our ability to make our own moral judgments. In fact, the opposite is true. Brave souls are willing to gain an understanding of someone's very different perspective without being forced to agree.

As believers who embody empathy, we are meant to be among the most unoffended, unthreatened, openhearted people on the planet. We are safe because Jesus led the way, never compromising truth.

Exercising our empathy muscle with those we don't "get" right away—and maybe never will—takes discipline. We aren't naturally drawn to discomfort, especially if there is no immediate extrinsic reward. But the return on investment is intrinsic; we grow on the inside. With practice and over time, any fear you have of "the other" will begin to drop away. Your brave soul will emerge more and more with each uncomfortable step.

BRAVE SOULS DON'T JUST HAPPEN

There are three ways to become better at something: practice every day, practice like it matters, and practice taking risks. When we focus on an activity, ritual, or liturgy, our repeated choices help turn empathy into a discipline, one that can help us become more able to know and to care for others. Choose empathy like it matters. How much we embody empathy will determine the amount of presence—God's presence and power—is released.

And don't be afraid to take risks. This is serious work, but not without joy—even in war zones. Just before we climbed Kilimanjaro, we visited our sisters in Congo, including Esperance. As we made our way into the cinderblock church, Lynne and I took great joy in seeing the faces of the sisters we had seen before. But instead of the fifteen women we had hoped for, almost forty had arrived. They had arrived to be seen, to be heard, to give their thumbprints. Their voices rose strong, their bodies, broken and healed, swayed and stomped and jumped, scattering hope to everyone who came into the room. Congo is full of suffering but also full of beauty, strength, and audacious joy. Brave souls open their hearts.

Too often we see only the suffering, the need, or the dark corners of life. Sometimes it feels as if risk-taking is just too risky. But what we often call failure is not failure at all because it's valuable for our growth and eventual success.

> *Too often we see only the suffering, the need, or the dark corners of life.*

Esperance and I stepped aside to talk while the climb sisters got to know the Congo sisters. We held hands again, like so many years before. She told me she was happy that her thumbprint was "famous," and I told her I was proud she went on to become a counselor.

Swiss-born psychiatrist and pioneer of the five stages of grief, Dr. Elisabeth Kübler-Ross wrote, "The most beautiful people I have known are those who have known defeat intimately, known suffering, known struggle, known loss, and have found their way out of the depths." Esperance remains an example for me. There are others too. Dorothy Day's legacy gives me hope still, almost every day. And Lynne has an appreciation, a sensitivity, and an understanding of pain in life that fills her with rare compassion, uncommon gentleness, and a genuine love for others.

These friends inspire me to carry on. I know you have friends who do the same.

But brave souls don't just happen. When they fall, they get up. In the face of disappointment and disillusionment, they rise from the ashes. Their failures are not wasted but are forged into an earthy grit, a hopeful commitment, a divine perseverance.

MAKE PRACTICE MATTER

In the end, I face only one question: Will I be a brave soul or not? The mountain taught me that either I'm willing to love like Jesus or I'm not really at all. As novelist Toni Morrison wrote, "Love is or it ain't. Thin love ain't love at all."

But staying connected to the heart and soul of Jesus, avoiding apathy and indifference, and fulfilling my call to care for others and understand their pain has turned out to be much harder than I thought. Laying down my reputation, my comfort, my agenda, and my judgment to love others as God loves them requires more than Kilimanjaro.

Empathy is not a one-off lesson, nor is it learned in a vacuum. We learn from and for others, and it always takes time and daily practice. Empathy is risky business, opening us up to seeing, hearing, and acting in new ways. Perspective-taking, empathetic listening, and peacemaking are its pathways. When pursued and practiced over and over again, they offer lessons most people rarely experience.

And these lessons are worth pursuing. Why? Because the way of empathy gives us the courage to embrace others in pain so healing can come. It gives us the wisdom to nurture hopes and inspire dreams toward growth and change. It gives us the kind of love that people crave, even if they don't know it.

Obviously I have empathy issues. The years I struggled with the classic hallmarks of high-functioning apathy were filled with a thin worldview, preoccupation with myself, and tendency to judge others. Now, there are days I feel three steps ahead, but there are still plenty of days when I feel two steps behind.

Yet I know and care more today than I did yesterday, and over time progress is progress. My teachers are those who are willing to climb with me, like Jesus did, not from a distance or removed, but connected.

We don't have to look alike. We don't have to agree. We don't have to have it all together. But we do have to love and, as Paul echoed Jesus' command, "Rejoice with those who rejoice; mourn with those who mourn. Live in harmony with one another. Do not be proud, but be willing to associate with people of low position. Do not think you are superior" (Romans 12:15-16).

These words strike me every time I read them. They resound with the countercultural command to be connected to others. Jesus called this perfect love. This kind of love doesn't just happen; it has to be learned and practiced. We learn in the climb, practice in the descent, just as Jesus did. "Son though he was, he learned obedience from what he suffered and, once made perfect, he became the source of eternal salvation for all who obey him" (Hebrews 5:8-9).

If I could make an imaginary leap into the backstory of the good Samaritan, I believe I could see many small moments when he'd choose to exercise—to practice, if you will—the humanizing of people. He'd see people in his home village refuse to give hospitality to Jews, and he'd quietly slip a skin of water to those asking for some. Maybe he'd traveled outside Samaria as a child, and seeing a Jewish boy just like him, they'd played together until adults noticed and spirited them away. He'd practice the many small acts of empathy that culminated in an act so extravagant that the story would be told by every generation since. I like to imagine later in Good Sam's life he'd know that the little acts of empathy in his early years had become models for those seeking to make a difference.

In my life, prayer has been the single most calming place for my panicky soul. For me, prayer is a form of practicing. When I press past a rush of adrenaline or burst beyond my stress to sit in front of God, I find not only peace but also real solutions to everyday obstacles. Imagination plays a huge role in knowing and caring for others, and prayers that genuinely make a difference require imagination. I wish I would have known this sooner in my life.

Even when my soul was slowly turning cold and gray with apathy, God sent empathy invitations to me. He whispered to me that though it felt like a descent, there would soon be a rising. Brave souls persevere, they practice, and they pray, until they rise stronger.

9

THE THUMBPRINT OF GOD

To love another person is to see the face of God.
Victor Hugo

I never would have believed that ferns—yes, the green feathery kind—would teach me so much. During our climb, I just passed them by. They were abundant, beautiful, and green—just like everything else in the foothills. It took Lynne's tears to help me see them—really see them. And when I did, everything came together for me.

We were a merry band those first few days. We chatted, we laughed, and we hiked in sync with each other until our bright but formidable guide, Lucy, taught us the magic words that would accompany us all the way to the top: *poly, poly*. Those words helped us to slow down, to measure our steps, to count the cost of energy given to talking, breathing, even gestures. As we slowed and quieted, we began to look around, some of us for the first time.

I'm so glad we did. Lynne had pulled off the trail and was standing by a grove of trees, gazing intently. As I came to her side, she took a deep breath and said, "I almost missed it, Belinda."

"Missed what?" I asked, straining to see what she saw. Was it a bug? A monkey? A brilliant bird? "The fern," she whispered, her sunglasses hiding tears. "My mom loved ferns. She would have loved these."

Lynne is one of the bravest souls I know. Her mother, Leah, had suddenly passed away just months before our trip. Lynne knew her mom would be proud she was climbing, especially because of who she was climbing in solidarity with. In her grieving, Lynne saw her mother in the intricate lace and curves of the flora.

I felt my throat tighten and my eyes sting as I looked. And something amazing happened. What I had not seen before, what had looked like only green bunches that we sped past toward our greater goal, suddenly became individual, unique banners of life weighed down by humidity in the still air. Some were curled up like hands, waiting to open. Some were browning and not long for this world. All were made up of the same repeated pattern of curves and edges emerging from a sturdy stem. The smallest section of leaf exactly mirrored the biggest part of the whole plant.

Now, ask me about coffee, and I can tell you a few things. Quiz me about Narnia, Sherlock Holmes, or *Doctor Who*, about raising boys or grading on a curve, about Thai food or what socks to wear with what sweater, and I think I could impress you. But I know very little about plants in general, and even less about ferns. Come to find out, Lynne and Leah were on to something big.

Ferns will blow your mind if you let them. There are close to fifteen thousand species. They self-reproduce (clever!) and can grow as small as a mouse or as tall as a tree. Not only are ferns the number one oxygen producing plant, they also absorb toxic chemicals in the air that can be fatal to us. Scientists say having a fern in your home can actually increase your life span.

But the truly mind-blowing part of ferns is this: they are fractals, the geometric result of repeating the same pattern over and over at a smaller and smaller scale. Fractals are the same big pattern shrinking every time it duplicates itself. Next time you're at a floral shop or walking in the woods, look at a fern. It is made up of the same feather-shaped pattern on a large and small scale. One single pattern repeats thousands of times, making up a whole fern frond. Experts say fractals can be divided and subdivided an infinite number of times. Infinite! It's so simple yet so complex. Ferns are creation unbounded for all to see. No wonder Lynne's mom loved them.

But fractals are not just found in ferns. They can be found everywhere. Pineapple for lunch? Fractal. Broccoli for dinner? Fractal. Stars? Yep. Snowflakes and shells, galaxies and lightning, peacock feathers, clouds, and crystals. Even mirror neurons are fractals. I couldn't hold back the tears when I realized mountains are fractals too.

But there is one fractal that stands above the rest. It is sublime, complete, and quintessentially unique yet exceptionally universal and powerful in its ability to recreate itself over and over: the human thumbprint. Each thumbprint—yours, mine, and each one collected at a bake sale, town hall meeting, conference, church, or school—is a tiny example of the infinite embodied in the finite. The fractal's geometry housed in a simple biometric identifier speaks to the infinite nature in each of us. The reason we climbed a mountain was for the idea of *infinite* love—empathy—embodied in a finite thumbprint. And our greatest hope is that thumbprints will beget thumbprints.

One million of them.

One fractal is sublime, complete, and quintessentially unique yet exceptionally universal and powerful in its ability to recreate itself over and over: the human thumbprint.

When mathematician Benoit Mandelbrot discovered fractals in the human body, including human fingerprints, he was so moved he called it the thumbprint of God. In them, he saw profound order in what seemed random: a chaotic, elegant design floating in a sea of chance. In the human thumbprint, he found meaning. "Order," he said, "doesn't come by itself."

And so, we end where our journey began: with a thumbprint. Your thumbprint is a testimony to God's infinite, fractal-like image in all of us and the image of God we form when stand together. God has chosen to make a mark on this world by leaving his mark in us. Call it God's design, the image of God, or simply God's thumbprint. I like to think of it as a soul print—his likeness pressed into the soft clay of our souls.

But as amazing and important as this is, bearing God's image is not an end in itself.

FROM KNOWING AND CARING TO DOING

Design always connotes a purpose—an elegant logic, a reason for being. God imprinted his image into our souls so that we can imprint his image onto the souls of others. This is our ultimate soul print, our mark.

Herein lies the crux of our journey together. Empathy must be given to something more than ourselves. If it isn't, it's not empathy at all. It remains aloof, an idea, mere rhetoric, a theory. Action must accompany our loftiest of thoughts, our most wrenching emotions, and our bravest commitments. Empathy without action undermines its very reason for being. The apostle James put it this way:

Do not merely listen to the word, and so deceive yourselves. Do what it says. Those who listen to the word but do not do what it says are like people who look at their faces in a mirror and, after looking at themselves, go away and immediately forget what they look like. But those who look intently into the perfect law that gives freedom and continue in it—not forgetting what they have heard but doing it—they will be blessed in what they do. (James 1:22-25)

When a journalist asked me if I was "still evangelical," I told him I had an uneasy relationship with that term because its meaning had changed. Now the word *evangelical* often means anything but "according to the teaching of the gospel of Christ, the good news." Evangelicals are perceived as exclusive and bigoted toward people unlike themselves.

The Bible says we will be known by our fruit, deeds, and actions, especially toward the vulnerable and disenfranchised. (See Matthew 25 and Isaiah 58, for example.) Our faith is proved by our actions. What separates the Christian God from all others is not ideas, theology, or words—as important as they are—but deeds done. Jesus of Nazareth was God dressed in human skin, donning the burden of pain and sorrow as well as pleasure and joy, each so integral to the human experience. Within his humanity he bore the image of his Father, the God of galaxies and ferns and fractals. And somewhere between heaven and earth, he slipped on thumbprints and left his mark on all of us, indelibly, faithfully, permanently. He demonstrated love for us—he didn't just talk about it or feel it—while we were yet sinners.

Our climb was an intimate lesson in what it means to understand how God's image, imprinted in us, is meant to be given away. Together we trekked through our motives, our sorrows, our successes, and our skills. We embraced the power of God's design for empathy in us. Together we made much headway in recognizing and calling out the soul print of others.

Empathy belongs to us. It's hardwired into us as part of God's design. It's learned through practical skills and sustained as a spiritual discipline. It's God's soul print in us, for us, and for others. We can learn to know and care. We can listen into the perspective of others. We can transform conflict, and the fruit that follows is abundant. We can freely choose to embody empathy in our day-to-day lives, pressing into the fear, pain, hope, and joy of others, and choosing to do something, to serve someone.

We are marked by God so we can make God's mark on others.

EMPATHY IN ACTION

My obsession with empathy was put to the test one winter morning just before Christmas. Advent is one of my favorite seasons, full of the ache, weight, and pressure of something about to be birthed. For more than a decade, I had given my passion and time toward ending violence against women in places such as Congo, South Sudan, and Syria. So naturally the #MeToo and #ChurchToo movements captured my attention. But they were deeply personal as well. Just as the movements were cresting across national media in 2017, I was taking courses in narrative therapy to better understand how I could serve victims of war violence.

Little did I know that these courses would impact me personally. While growing up, I had experienced a handful of incidents that ranged from harassment to manipulation to sexual violence, but I had repressed those memories. My own story was part of the #MeToo story. With the help of a circle of trusted counselors, I was able to walk through them—and oceans of fear, anger, and tears. Thank God for a redemption that is raw, tangible, and real. I needed it—and still need it—far more than I knew.

One of the most painful realizations in these heady days of speaking truth to power, is how the church is prone to be silent when a woman experiences harassment, assault, or all-out violence, especially when the violence occurred in the church itself. Why would a church that purports to follow the One who reached across barriers to talk to the woman who was bleeding, who offered a Samaritan woman "living water," and who disarmed a mob set on stoning an adulteress, remain silent on violence against women?

> *Why would a church that purports to follow the One who reached across barriers to talk to the woman who was bleeding, who offered a Samaritan woman "living water," and who disarmed a mob set on stoning an adulteress, remain silent on violence against women?*

I was working through a question: What does empathy look like for women who come forward to tell their stories only to face dismissal, gossip, degradation, and even accusation? I called our trusted, long-time friend, Rev. Lisa Sharon Harper, to ask what we could do together to speak up for our sisters. Her answer is seared in my memory: "Belinda, this is possible, and now is the moment. History has never seen a denominationally broad, racially diverse, global movement of women standing together for women. If you are serious about inviting everyone—and I mean everyone—I am in."

After I hung up, I took to my knees, thanking God for making a way forward. Nine days later, after countless sleepless hours, hundreds of phone calls, and other work done by a small army of dedicated women elders, theologians, leaders, advocates, activists, community organizers, directors, writers, speakers, and—above all—sisters, #SilenceIsNotSpiritual was born. We wrote a statement inviting the church to break the silence on violence against women, launching it during Christmas week. We began with more than one hundred and fifty signatories, leaders from many faith traditions and racial and cultural backgrounds, each with her own story. In those early days, we were gaining more than a thousand signatures a day. We've launched in Brazil with plans to launch in Nigeria soon.

But this is only one example of empathy in action. My friend Idelette McVicker is a brave woman; her words and life are lethal to injustice, apathy, and the empathy-hindering voices of shame. She is a mother of three and, in her own words, "a restaurant wife who loves Jesus, justice, and living juicy." She is an Afrikaner born and raised in South Africa during the apartheid years, which both "wrecked" her and seeded a deep longing for a more free, reconciled, and just world. Her life journey took her to Taiwan where she drove a purple scooter, wrote for a daily newspaper, and discovered Jesus at a table full of women. In 1999, she moved to Vancouver, Canada, with her husband, where she founded and launched *SheLoves Magazine*, a global community of women "who want to know and experience freedom, justice and transformation, for ourselves and others." An empathetic mission statement if there ever was one!

Idelette is, in her words, "called to pay attention to where women are missing in the world." One week after the tragedy of 9/11, she sat shoulder-to-shoulder with more than fifteen thousand women at the Houston Astrodome where she watched a video called "Tears: Women in Afghanistan." The words of an Afghan sister were a wake-up call for Idelette, who wrote, "We need the women of the world to come looking for us; we need the hope that someone would come looking for us when we're missing." Idelette said,

[The video] shook me at the core of my being, because I could hear the cry of a sister on the other side of the world.

Truth is, I had not seen her. I did not go looking for her. I had been wrapped up in my own story of freedom. But coming face to face with the reality of the oppression of women worldwide changed my life forever. I wanted to go look for and stand with the women who were missing in our world.

And she did. Following the lead of her indigenous sisters, Idelette is learning to advocate with and for indigenous women and also raise awareness of missing and murdered indigenous women and girls in Canada. While it's difficult to identify the total number who are missing or murdered, we know that indigenous women are *three and half times* more likely to experience violence than non-indigenous women.

Learning to ask the right questions is a beginning. We need to ask hard, uncomfortable questions like, *Why do our sisters go missing?* and, *What systems make it possible for them to go missing in the first place?* "A part of us will always be missing, until there is justice and visibility and acknowledgement of those who are missing," Idelette said. "A part of our voice cannot rise until their voices rise." And because there has been little to no response or recourse to date, we are left to ask with our indigenous sisters everywhere, "Do we know? Do we care? Will we do something to find our sisters? *Will we tell the world?*"

Not everyone needs to climb a mountain. My friend Lynne's advice to simply ask, "What is mine to do?" is a brilliant place to start. Maybe pioneering a campaign or joining a cause seems overwhelming. Don't worry; empathy in action need not be complex. Maybe you can reach across cultural boundaries by inviting an immigrant or refugee family out for lunch. Or the next time you see a homeless person, stop and ask for her name and listen to her story, should she want to talk. Even a truthful social media hashtag, standing up for the dignity of another facing sexism, racism, or another form of systematic bullying, is empathy showing up. Sometimes empathy in action begins with nothing more than a simple hopeful word when everyone else is complaining or cynical. We can all start now, as we are, where we are.

A few small actions might take you on a surprising journey. Next thing you know, you may just find yourself in the company of superheroes.

THE WONDER WOMEN OF SYRIA

Few people would question that superhero Wonder Woman is a woman of action. When the film by that name, starring Gal Gadot, broke box office records worldwide, several countries in the Middle East banned it, and protestors in Austin, Texas, picketed women-only showings. Tribe was on full display as one American news anchor complained that the heroine wasn't "American enough."

As the world debated the merits and missed opportunities of *Wonder Woman*, I traveled to the Beqaa Valley in Lebanon, a stone's throw from the city of Damascus at the Syrian border, to interview the real wonder women of Syria: refugee women who have experienced inconceivable suffering and who fight every day to overcome it.

Zada definitely did not look like Wonder Woman. Yet as we talked, she revealed herself to be far from mild mannered. As she pushed back her head covering, she shifted uncomfortably in her chair. She was eight months pregnant, a refugee, and had just arrived at the border. I was uncomfortable for her. Shaking her head, she pressed the puffy fingers of her right hand firmly into what little waist she had left as her baby inside kicked. A *finjaan* (handleless coffee cup) balancing on her swollen belly swayed with each kick. "She will be strong," Zada said, grinning at me as she moved her cup to avoid a spill, her smile dissolving into a deadly seriousness. "We need her to be strong," she said.

My quest to find the wonder women of the world who had survived the terror of living in war zones grew out of a deepening desire to hear the voices of women rise from the ashes born on that Mother's Day many years ago. Over the past five years, I've interviewed almost a hundred women who call the place they live a war zone. The vast majority of them are mothers. Many are grandmothers. All of them are daughters. But no matter what their status, each of them knows what it means to love like a mother. These women are the world's hidden heroes—the real wonder women.

Zada now lives ten minutes from the Lebanese border of her homeland, Syria. Her story, like so many, is one of fleeing violence and devastation, overcoming insurmountable odds to protect her kids, clinging fiercely to the hope that the children of Syria can have a future. The makeshift camps nestled in Beqaa Valley, where the poppy fields were in full bloom, were filled with ten-by-twelve-foot rooms, tarped against rain and snow from the recent winter months. Tens of thousands of Syrians call these camps home.

Since 2011, the entire population of Lebanon has increased by half as they opened their gates to more than two million people fleeing the civil war. I was sobered to the core when I learned that the vast majority of those fleeing are women and children.

Zada had five daughters; only four are alive now. At age thirty-six, she seems haunted as she tells us of her daughter Rasha. She would have been a little more than one year old if she had lived. Doctors told the family that Rasha had a hole between the lower ventricle walls of her heart. Sometimes Rasha would turn a bright blue and even pass out. She wasn't getting enough oxygen to her blood. In the United States, many infants who have surgery for this grow up to live normal lives. But your chances plummet when you're a child in a war.

Medical care in refugee camps can feel like a luxury item, so when a doctor offered to do the open-heart surgery for $10,000

(US) in cash, though it was an astronomical sum, Zada said yes. Surrounded by both refugee and local women, Rasha received the surgery. She fought for her life, but the doctor said she just "didn't make it" and turned over the baby's body to Zada and her husband—no questions allowed.

As a refugee, Zada was left with no recourse and no way to know what happened to her daughter. She turned to her sisters. She had lost her home, her country, and now her daughter. She was at risk of losing her soul. What she needed was empathy and great courage. She needed to be found.

The weight of war on mothers is more than just physical. As I talked to women at the camps, it was easy to see evidence of trauma at epidemic levels. Up to half of all women and girls living in the prolonged, extreme-stress situation of the refugee camps in Lebanon experience depression associated with physical and mental violence. Feelings of abandonment and deep grief accompany their trauma. "There was no hope left in Syria for us. So we fled," whispered Amira, mother of two. At age thirty-six, she holds a degree in Arabic literature, something she and her children are very proud of. She hopes someday to put her degree to use in helping the children from her conflicted homeland.

As we talked, Amira's bright eyes grew dark as she remembered living in a war zone. "War arrived in our home, and we had no heat, no gas, no food, no water," she said. Amira recalled the first time she fed her children spoiled vegetables and moldy bread from a trash bin. She remembers avoiding the gunfire as she ran back to her apartment with the food. Caught in the height of battle for "the capital of the revolution," Amira and her children were targets for ruthless rooftop snipers.

She and her husband waited out the nearly four months of fierce antigovernment clashes that left more than 1,500 dead. Then they fled for Lebanon. "As Christians, we knew we were in danger, and there were many good Muslims that helped us escape the city," she said. Though Lebanon opened its doors to her family, their suffering continued as her husband coped with the trauma through heavy drinking, disappearing for long periods, and finally vanishing all together.

> *"As Christians, we knew we were in danger, and there were many good Muslims that helped us escape the city."*
> AMIRA

"I was again alone," Amira said, patting her chest with her hand, as if calming a small child. Her hands shook slightly. She insisted that faith, prayer, and a hope in a loving God kept her from despairing altogether. Until that day, she had supported her children doing whatever was necessary to make sure they were fed and in some form of school. She had begged help from family, sold produce on the streets, and most recently, began working in a local school helping Muslim refugees to assimilate and heal as they learn.

She too seeks healing and says she is learning to forgive in the midst of her greatest sadness: realizing she and her children can never go back home again to Homs, her city in Syria. As a mother raising young children completely alone in a new country, home is the only place Amira wants to be. But home no longer exists.

FACING INDIGNITIES

The fear of being forgotten is very real for these women. As many as one-fourth of all Syrian refugee women find themselves, like Amira, resource strapped and feeling abandoned while trying to take care of traumatized children. Well over 70 percent of Syrian refugees worldwide live in grinding poverty, trying to make it on less than two dollars a day in insecure dwellings with limited food access. Many of these mothers say they aren't safe; some never leave their tent.

The stigma of being a stranger at a time when Syrian refugees are seen as backward and simple robs these women of what little dignity and honor they have. Many lament the way they are treated. They are sexually and economically harassed. They are forced to endure slanders and slurs. In Zahle, many of the women who live on informal refugee plots must go out to the fields with their young daughters to pick potatoes and other produce to "pay the rent" their landlords demand. If they do not pick, they cannot stay. Or they can "pay another way." There are widespread reports of men illegally "marrying" young girls, paying bride prices to their cash-strapped fathers or brothers, only to turn around and leave them weeks later with a divorce settlement for "services rendered."

Myriam knows firsthand the indignity refugee women face. She and her husband fled Syria with two boys at the beginning of the war. Now she has only one. "When the war started, you didn't know who was against you—it was a mess," she said. She was a respected teacher, her husband had a good job, and her two sons enjoyed their school. All this changed during the siege of Myriam's home city, which quickly became ISIL-held territory. In the midst of fleeing from city to city to find refuge, her oldest son, Hani, was killed by mortar fire. As she told her story, she glanced up at the photo of him hanging on her wall, explaining how snipers kept her from going to him as he lay in the hospital. It still haunts her that her son died alone.

Myriam's traumatized family eventually fled to Lebanon, experiencing illness, homelessness, and poverty. Though she has years of experience as a certified teacher, she now picks up the trash that students drop on the floor as a part-time school cleaner. She says students chide her as they drop a dirty tissue on the floor and say, "You have to pick it up. You serve us now." Yet she clings to her dignity, remaining strong, beautiful, and resilient enough to stand up to the dehumanization the majority of refugees face on every front.

> *Students chide her as they drop a dirty tissue on the floor and say, "You have to pick it up. You serve us now."*

Zada, Amira, Myriam, and so many like them have stood strong in the face of fear, poverty, trauma, and harassment. Nothing unifies them more than their hopes and dreams for their children. According to the United Nations, more than eighty thousand babies have been born abroad to the refugees of Syria. Lebanon is quickly becoming home to an entire generation of Syrian babies, a generation at risk of being abandoned or lost altogether to disease, poverty, and the harshness of life in the camps. They feel the weather acutely, and tents can be twice as hot or twice as cold as anywhere else, exposing babies to extreme heat and cold, causing them to suffer greatly. Infant deaths to hypothermia and heat exhaustion continue to rise. Food rations are meager, and attempting to create a balanced diet for a pregnant mother or a growing child is close to impossible. And as in Zada's case, medical access for safe deliveries and follow-up child-maternal health care are not only complicated to receive but also very expensive.

FINDING HOPE

Yet in this crucible of conflict, the refugees of Beqaa Valley have a reason to hope, a reason to believe they and their children have been found. These wonder women, like their superhero counterpart, take the blows, absorb them, and turn them into strength to fight the good fight. Take Izdihar, mother of two, and founder of Together for the Family, a local nonprofit serving refugees. Izdihar, a Syrian who has seen years of war herself, loves nothing more than bringing diapers, vitamins, formula, medicine, seasonal clothes, and blankets to the mothers of newborns and growing babies—and, as in her case, financial help for medical expenses.

"This one is my favorite," she chirps as she scoops up a beautiful, healthy baby girl with cheeks like small apples, carrying her as we visit the roughed-out tent camp. I quickly get the feeling she said this about every baby she has ever met and meant it for each one entirely.

Speaking in Arabic, Izdihar extolls the virtues of child-maternal mental and physical health, trauma reduction, counseling, and medical support as she helps mothers procure bags of socks and toys for the sweltering summer and extra-warm woolly onesies with matching hats and scarves for the harsh winters. Today, these wide-eyed little ones cry, feed, coo, and gurgle as women of all faiths and backgrounds bow their heads to pray together, each respecting the intimate bond being formed between each other beyond political affiliation, religion, culture, or circumstance.

Those at Together for the Family have all suffered. They have all feared. Some were considered sworn enemies, while others were considered untouchable outsiders. Yet all their little ones were born in exile. And now each possesses the greatest secret weapon against fear they have ever known: the hope hidden in babies. As mothers, these women see themselves in each other and the hope for a future in each other's children. No matter where they are from or where they hope to go, the power of empathy makes them stronger, braver, and even fearless at times.

As a little girl, I wanted to be just like Wonder Woman, able to absorb blow after blow with my indestructible bracelets and rescue the day, emerging even stronger than before. As I grew up, I began to notice something about the plethora of superhero movies, comics, and binge-worthy TV series. Nestled between the rising conflict, the dire straits, and the shock and awe is a moment when the superhero confronts her greatest fear—and overcomes it. The same is true for these mothers. They don't ask for pity. They barely ask for help. But the depth of pain and sorrow they feel is real. And very much like the superheroes of our dreams, what they desire is stunningly simple and similar across history, geography, culture, and socioeconomic boundaries: to be given the chance to bring hope where hope is needed most.

Wonder Woman may be banned, picketed, and debated, but these women will continue their silent, thankless heroism by surviving day by day with Herculean strength. Their hope demands it, and sometimes their faith does too—for their children, their families, their sisters. It's what heroes do. Empathy doesn't just talk; it *does*.

Zada, Amira, Myriam, Izdihar: we see you, brave souls. You give us hope.

EMPATHY AS WORSHIP

There is one more lesson. We know the purpose of empathy is to love—genuinely love—our neighbor, our God, and ourselves. When we try to love with words only, our intentions fall flat because we do not act. Empathy without deeds is mere rhetoric.

But the image of God in us, imprinted so that we can imprint the nature of God into others, is for another reason. There is an ultimate Other, one we can listen to, take the viewpoint of, take action on behalf of, and authentically love. All we have learned can be applied to God.

Empathy for God? Really?

Yes. The ancient spiritual discipline of holy empathy, not for the faint of heart, will lead us to a radical, brave love for God and a life of glorifying and enjoying him forever. Empathy is an act of worship.

Have you ever heard the prayer "Break my heart, God, with the things that break yours"? Empathy for God. Or what about the phrase "God became like us so we can become like him"? Empathy for God. Or think about the verse "I no longer live, but Christ lives in me" (Galatians 2:20). Christ is in us, his life, his Spirit, his sorrow, his joy, all coursing through our veins. Yep, empathy for God. "We have the mind of Christ," the apostle Paul wrote (1 Corinthians 2:16). Empathy—heart, mind, and soul.

When we willingly see others and ourselves as God sees us, we come to know God's character, training our eyes to see what is unseen and eternal. When we know God, we become like God, bravely recognizing his image in others.

Throughout my journey it was in my challenges I felt closest to God. In my most difficult moments, I heard God the clearest, most often in the voice of others. During the moments I was brave, risking the vulnerability required when embodying empathy, God showed up. When we weep, God weeps. When we rejoice, God rejoices. When we stand, God stands. Our minds become God's mind. Our hands become God's hands.

May God establish the mark you make as you courageously take the world into your hands, pressing your thumb into the clay lives of others. God invites us to overcome, take risks, do great things, and love powerfully, extravagantly, audaciously.

Always take courage in a world gone mad, brave soul.

You may just save us all.

ACKNOWLEDGMENTS

"Show me your friends," says an old Mexican proverb, "and I will show you who you are." If the wisdom of this saying proves true, I am one of the bravest women alive. It was for you, brave souls, that I wrote. And rewrote. And rewrote again. I pray that what you find here brings you hope.

First, thank you, Esperance. Your mandate changed my life and someday I pray, our whole world. I will forever be grateful to you, bravest of souls. And thank you to ALL my survivor sisters for telling your stories to the world. You have made your mark on me.

Thank you, Stephan. You loved me from day one (literally!) and have made me better, stronger, and braver ever since. Thank you, Joshua, for patiently listening every time I showed up at your door to "read a sentence" that inevitably turned into reading a whole chapter. Thank you for sharing your old-soul wisdom so generously. And Caleb, thank you for always giving me that perfectly timed hug, the exact words to make me brave again. You always get me. The three of you are the men in my life, and your empathy toward women and their stories, and your belief in their bravery give me hope for the future of our world.

To Shayne, Kimberly, and Inge-Lise, the dedicated, talented, and generous directors at One Million Thumbprints. May the mountains we climb together be many and miraculous. And thank you to our wonderful, patient, and long haul board members: Robert Maupin, Suby Wildman, and Kostas Kotopoulos.

Thank you, my sister Kilimanjaro climbers. I count our journey together as the most important in my life. Your brave souls have breathed oxygen into my soul—and if anyone in the world knows how valuable oxygen is, it is you! It is my joy to honor you here with our story, deeply connected and rooted in holy empathy. Oh, and yes—I would do it again with you in a heartbeat. You dear ones—Ruth, Joy Beth, Kim, Jen, Chelsea, Laura, Brenda, Kris, Krista, Chessy, and Leia—you are the very definition of BRAVE SOULS.

And to my dear friend Lynne. You once said to me that "in the space of the Spirit, grief and lament need not cancel out joy and hope." I keep your words close—inhaling hope and exhaling pain. And in that hope, I dream of the new mountains God will call us to climb for the sake of peace and for the One who loves and believes in women. Thank you for always protecting, always trusting, always hoping, and always persevering. You love so well, sister.

And to my dear friend Alyce, I like who I became the day we decided to be the best of friends. You are a learner, a leader, and a lioness. I love your beautiful girls—Karissa, Lorra, Annika, and Brielle—to the summit and back.

Many thanks to our dear friends who love above and beyond the call of duty, David and Tina Lippiatt and the team at WE International, for all you did to get us to the top! David—mountains suit you, brother, keep climbing! Tina, I know your prayers change many bad things to good. Thank you, sister. And to you, Jay and Judy, Jared, Jillian and Brett, Tim and Terri, and cousins Jeff and Tricia—friendships are made for adventures in doing good!

A mountain of thanks to the all-star African Walking Company. Each member of the team was our coach, our guide, our cheerleader, our brother, our sister. May you prosper and grow to one day hire and train the first all-Tanzanian, all-woman's guide team. And when that happens, count us in for round two!

Thank you, my sister Lebanon-Mountain climbers. You are the most brilliant, empathetic group of BACL's I have ever met. I love you Peggy, Sandi, Lyric, Demi, Inge-Lise, Tracy, Katy, Nicol, Zinnia. And to you, Ruth and Alyce—for saying yes, once again.

And to Team Vanden Bos—Curtis and Susan. Climbing two volcanoes in Mexico to raise awareness for Syrian refugees is a shining example of the brave souls you are. Thank you for knowing, for caring, and for acting so beautifully.

My dear friend and sister Izdihar—every day you inspire me to be better, to do better, and to take the "very big risks" of loving God by loving others through giving it all away. Thank you, Kassis family, for taking in the Baumans as your own.

I am grateful to those who sustained us as we traveled the globe. For us, you and your families will always be "home." Andy, Sunita, Gabe, Addie, and goddaughter Asha—your gift of welcome, acceptance and support never fails, and we love you for it! To Bill and Tara Haley, Cyprian and Zeburia Nkiriyumwami Nicolas and Elsie Hitimana, John Paul and Clementine Ndagijimana, Karen and Peter Schulze, Chuck and Sue Duby. John and Roanna, Malia and Kennedy, Branden and Jessica Pustejovsky, Rob and Wanda Gailey—each one of you breathe brave back into our souls. Thank you for the years and years of generosity, hospitality, love, and care.

Thank you to the incredible team at IVP. Jeff Crosby, your empathy toward me over breakfast is the reason we hold these words in our hands today. Cindy Bunch, my brilliant editor, your empathy toward me over lunch is the reason these words are so much better than I ever thought they could be. And to Helen Lee and Lori Neff, your empathy toward me over breakfasts, lunches, and dinners is the reason these words shine for the world to see! I am humbled and honored to have worked with such world-class people.

I am beyond grateful for the embodied theology and friendship of Lisa Sharon Harper, and the brilliant people at Freedom Road, and Emily Nielsen Jones and the leaders of Imago Dei. The world needs you now like it never has, my friends. Thank you for fearlessly answering the call.

I am beyond grateful to each of the voices who influenced my journey from apathy to empathy to action. Without you, your words of truth and life and trust would be buried in a drawer, feared or forgotten. You brought the brave by speaking it, writing it, preaching it, producing it, singing it, being it —JoAnne Lyon, Abigale Disney, Cheryl Bridges Johns, Carolyn Custis James, Kelley Nikondeha, Judy Douglass, Max and Kate Finburg, Ali Noorani, Michael and Melissa Wear, Ashlee and Delwin Eiland, Shannon Dingle, Craig Stewart and the good people of the Warehouse, Gabe and Jeanette Salguero, Chi Chi Okwu, Paul and Christy Borthwick, Mimi Haddad, Ken and Tamara Wytsma, Don and Deyon Stephens, Dr. Gary and Susan Parker and our Mercy Ships family, Robyn Afrik, Dr. Sandra Morgan and the Global Center for Women and Justice, Matthew Soerens, Austin Channing Brown, Lisa-Jo Baker, Logan Wolfram, Amena Brown, Shauna Niequist, Idelette McVicker and the dangerous women she leads, Katelyn Beaty, Diana Oosterwyk, Beth Birmingham, Jenny Yang, Mae Cannon, Muriele and Duane Elmer, Zach Hoag, Greg and Kit Elmer, Scott Buresh, Steve Wiens, Rev. Darren Harkins, John and Susan Yeats, Father Michael White, Steve and Sarah Carter, Josh and Natalie Salminen, Josh and Michelle Garrells, Ted and Kellie Haddock, the brilliant

Micah Bournes, and the many brave souls who risk truth telling and peacemaking every day.

To Kathy Khang and Sandra Van Opstal, thank you for expecting more of me than I ever thought I could live out. You show me what brave looks like every day. May there be much fasting and feasting together in our future, my sisters.

Deep thanks to the wonderful people who cheered as I climbed this mountain, and even more importantly, stood by me in the descent—a true friend does both! Thanks to the 2016 Chaplegate XC Team, 1MT interns Christopher Niccolini, Caroline Bair, and Madalyn Ames, and the brilliant students and friends making their mark at Grand Rapids Christian High School—you are brave souls already and give me hope for the future! I'm beyond grateful for Todd Deatherage and the peacemakers at Telos, Mark and Vickie Reddy and all at The Justice Conference, all the brilliant and brave souls of World Relief, Susan Shadid and Elie Pritz at The Jerusalem School, Fred Smith and family at The Gathering, Ed and Donna Stetzer, and Laurie Nichols at The Billy Graham Center, Robert Gallagher and Scott Moreau at Wheaton College, and Evvy Campbell. To those at Covenant College who formed my mind and heart integrally—Dr. Derek Halvorson, Brian Fikkert, Steve Corbett, Russ Mask, Becky Pennington, Rebecca Dodson, Jack Beckman, Jay Green, Phil Horton, Stephen Kaufman, Bill Davis, and Bruce Young. To the wonderful women of Red Tent Living—thank you for leading and redefining not only femininity, but faithfulness. And to Red Bud Writers—thank you for the audacious generosity of brain cells, encouragement, and spirit. I am proud to be a Bud! And finally, to our long-time friends Rob and Crystal Morris, Steve and Jamie Martin, and all those at LOVE 146 who press into the beauty of defiant hope!

Thank you, Mom, for always fostering curiosity and courage in me, whether trying new flips or trying new books, you made me believe I could succeed. And thank you, Dad, for always having the last word, especially when those words were "love you most. . . ." Thank you, Phil and Chris, Katie and David and family, for being beautiful examples of risk takers willing to leave a loving mark in difficult places. And my dear sister, Roxanne, your survivor soul glows with grace. My beloved Mom and Dad Bauman, and my sisters-in-love Brenda (selah), Pam and Rita, Marcy and Lawrence, and all the nieces and nephews—thank you for wrapping your arms around me and calling me Bauman.

And finally, thank you, dear God, for teaching us to love one another. Your law is love and your gospel is peace, and we know you are breaking every chain, for the slave is our sister and in your name all violence shall cease.

May ever word written here bring you glory.

APPENDIX A

REFLECTING ON YOUR EMPATHETIC LISTENING SKILLS

Empathetic listening is knowing and caring about what someone is saying, both verbally and nonverbally. It is listening according to Jesus' rule of love—that is, loving *as* he loved. Empathetic listening pays careful and sustained attention to what is being said in a variety of situations. Listening is a skill that is hardwired into humans at birth and can be developed into empathetic listening with practice.

Take a moment to reflect on your conversations with friends, your spouse, family members, coworkers, clients, or other staff. On the following chart, rate each remark as truthfully as possible by circling the best adjective—*often*, *sometimes*, *rarely*, or *never*—to help you reflect on your empathetic listening skills. If you're brave, ask a trusted friend, spouse, family member, or coworker to answer these questions about you. Then compare your answers. The Listening Reflection can be used within groups, departments, or project teams to start dialogues around listening capacity.

	OFTEN	SOMETIMES	RARELY	NEVER
After a conversation or discussion, I have a clear memory of what information was covered.	●	○	○	●
I concentrate on giving a speaker my undivided attention.	●	○	○	●
I resist composing my response in my head before the speaker is done.	●	○	○	●
I try to hold on to my thoughts rather than jump into a conversation.	●	○	○	●
I try not to give my opinion until the speaker is finished speaking.	●	○	○	●
I resist other activities such as checking my phone or scanning the room when listening to a lecture or having a conversation.	●	○	○	●
I resist finishing the sentences of others in my head or out loud.	●	○	○	●
I am willing to check in with the person I'm speaking with to make sure my understanding is correct.	●	○	○	●
I nod and make other gestures to show I'm interested in the conversation.	●	○	○	●
I concentrate on what the speaker is not saying as much as what they are saying.	●	○	○	●
In a conflict, I respectfully, rather than defensively, present my opinions.	●	○	○	●
If bored or uninterested in a conversation, I work hard to refocus quickly when I drift.	●	○	○	●
I can listen to others discuss their opinions without feeling that my own is threatened.	●	○	○	●
I am uncomfortable speaking over someone, even if I think I know what they're going to say.	●	○	○	●

Now what? Empathy has the potential to turn your life upside down. This may not happen all at once, but it will certainly surprise you. As you begin experiencing the skills of empathy—perspective-taking, empathetic listening, and peacemaking—let your community, whether next door or across the world, lift you up as you climb your mountain.

Many of these questions have served to reveal things in my own practice that need attention or continued reinforcement. I've had to recognize my difficulty with talking over people and interrupting their sentences by either finishing them or starting new ones. I know, right? Awful. In recognizing my weakness, I have actively been seeking a reset.

Though this may be hard to hear, asking why you do the things you do is key. I feared forgetting that point I wanted to make if I had to wait until other people made theirs. Yes, even now as I write this I recognize it was all about competing for my idea, my words, my win. I asked God to forgive me of my pride and to give me a clear understanding of who I was. My honesty helped me become more self-aware. I was able to lean into new paths of vulnerability and begin to change.

Becoming a better listener can often feel like an uphill climb, but the summit is worth it. Responding can take many forms, such as checking in with a trusted friend. Sometimes a quick internal high-five when you do well and a simple apology when you slip can help move you through the change process.

EMPATHY MAPPING: PUTTING IT ALL TOGETHER

Finding a brave soul is like finding a diamond. Much like diamonds, souls have to be mined. Mining these gems requires searching for them, and a treasure map can show us the path. Along the way, we discover diamonds in ourselves too.

Some souls are easy to find, having been made useful and steadfast by time and suffering, or polished to a brilliant beauty by surviving and overcoming trauma. Others are buried deep in the bedrock of circumstances and limitations. Because each person is created in the image of God, each soul is a divine invitation. The way of empathy provides a map to help you discover the diamond in each individual you encounter. As in real mining, discovering a diamond requires perseverance, patience, and careful attention. Most diamonds are found deep beneath the earth's surface and need to be excavated. On average, more than twenty tons of rock must be processed to procure just one diamond. Determining the value of a diamond requires crushing, cleaving, shaping, and polishing. In the end, the value of a diamond is decided by the internal beauty and strength magnified by its many facets.

And so it is with souls.

The individual facets on a diamond are what bring both light and clarity to the whole gem. Recognizing the value of souls is a skill we access by learning the way of empathy. This is very similar to holding up a diamond to the light and gazing through one facet to gain understanding of its true value.

The way of empathy has the potential to reveal the hidden qualities in every soul. Being trained in perspective-taking, empathetic listening, and peacemaking can first prepare *us* to understand *others*. When our hearts are prepared, we can reveal *others* to *us*. Consider the Empathy Diamond figure below as a kind of map, where the lower facets are skills we learn to help us appreciate what is then revealed by the top facets—the aspects of life that make us truly human: what brings us pain and fear, what we love, hope for, and rejoice over. Think about the colleague at work you just can't figure out, your emerging teenager who spends more time behind closed doors than out in the open, the relative who picks a fight every Thanksgiving, or the local leader who continues to confound your sensibilities.

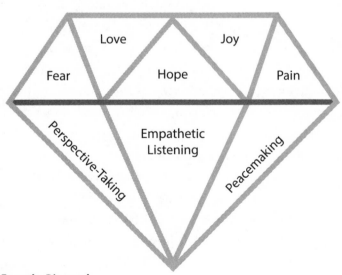

The Empathy Diamond

GETTING PRACTICAL

Stephan and I once asked our brilliant friend, Rev. Dr. JoAnne Lyon, the first woman general superintendent for the Wesleyan Church, her best advice for poverty alleviation. "Don't ask people what they need," was her immediate response. "Ask them what they hope for."

While everyone is unique, certain core motivations, experiences, and desires are common to all of us. What do we worry about or fear? What pain have we encountered or are we encountering? Where do we find joy? What do we dream about? What do we hope for? Following the way of empathy involves three stages, starting at the point of a diamond soul and working its way up through each facet.

First, consider who and why. This diamond soul belongs to someone or a group of someones. Who are they? Why do you want to understand them? Define your primary purpose for empathizing with this person or group. What outcome do you hope for? To initiate a new relationship? To gain understanding? To close a narrative gap? To influence a decision? To transform conflict? Unless you're clear on your purpose, you will be tossed about by every wind of strong emotion or wave of external circumstance.

Second, engage your empathy skills. This stage has one purpose: using the three empathy skills discussed in chapters four, five, and six to prepare to understand others. Increasing our ability to be receptive to human nuance, allowing us to open up and personally change as well, helps us to see people as far more than mere categories, statistics, or stereotypes.

Skill 1. Perspective-taking. At its most basic level, perspective-taking is jumping the gap between "my here" and "your there." When we start caring about the point of view of others, we're more likely to consider their perspectives, increasing our physical, attributional, and conceptual awareness through these three steps:

- *Humanize.* Drop the "me versus you" attitude; instead, send signals that the other person is valuable and valued.

- *Mind the gap.* Recognize that both you and she have different contexts. Acknowledge that there is a gap between the two and work to close it through observing and orienting.

- *Shift your perspective.* Empower, don't limit. Consider the stakes for her personally and offer possibilities for making her situation better.

Skill 2. Empathetic listening. Empathetic listening seeks to do two things: connect mind and heart with the person speaking and understand before being understood by listening into others rather than listening at them. Follow these steps.

- *Listen before you listen.* Pre-listening is paying attention to the noise that inhibits your ability to listen.

- *Discover the person you think you know.* Listen to discover who he really is and what he really is trying to say. Lean into rather than "listen at." Learn to hear his words and to "read the air" around him.

- *Be vulnerable.* Vulnerability requires personal risk, humility, and mutuality in our listening.

Skill 3. Peacemaking. Embrace opposition as an opportunity. Change requires us to define our tribe by who we are, not by who we are against. Every conflict or collision yields choices that can lead to change. Follow these steps.

- *Confront the conflict.* Conflict is normal, no matter how uncomfortable, and it can become a beautiful collision.

- *Make your choice.* When we embrace conflict, we make choices from a heart of war, which entrenches stereotypes and disconnection, or from a heart of peace, which encourages relationships and the pursuit of change.

- *Become the change.* Our choices allow us to become peacemakers by restoring relationships in our communities and our world.

Third, embody empathy. After having done the hard work of perspective-taking, listening, and peacemaking, we're ready to experience another person through five essential human facets: fear, love, hope, joy, and pain. As we do, we remain in the posture of presence and vulnerability, open to our own change and remembering the context as we ask the following questions about the person or people we're considering as well as ourselves:

- What do you fear?

- What causes you pain?

- What do you hope for?

- Who do you love?

- What brings you joy?

When we embody empathy, our lives become billboards for God, envoys of change, and vessels of restoration. We can be catalysts and ambassadors for reconciliation (2 Corinthians 5:20), healing a conflict, empowering change, or unearthing lost dreams.

As you record your responses along the way, cluster them around similar ideas and concepts. What will emerge is a greater sense of confidence that you "get" the person you are seeking to love. You will better understand the context she is living in. You will know if you have succeeded as you feel in your gut a growing assurance you have honored the *imago Dei* in this person, no matter how complex or simple, kind or difficult she may be.

QUESTIONS FOR PERSONAL REFLECTION OR GROUP DISCUSSION

PART ONE: WHY EMPATHY CAN SAVE US

1. In certain pockets of our culture, the topic of empathy is increasingly popular. There is even empathy marketing. But empathy as a practice is declining drastically, creating the empathy gap we're experiencing today. Belinda suggests that her empathy gap was filled with a Christian-veneered indifference, or *apathy*—literally, "without feeling"—that left her disconnected from the people around her. Others fill their gap with passive-aggressive *antipathy* or culturally acceptable surface *sympathy*. Where do you see the results of the empathy gap in our communities today? In our institutions? In our churches? Where have you fallen into the empathy gap? What "pathies" have you filled your gap with?

2. Esperance gave Belinda a glimpse of hope in one of the most difficult places in the world. In her "beautiful collision," Belinda witnessed Esperance's overcoming of insurmountable odds through the disruptive force of empathy, which Belinda defined as *knowing and caring to the point of action*. What are some of our culture's most difficult places? What are some of your most difficult places? How might the power of empathy help overcome some of your own dysfunctional cycles?

3. Read Matthew 7:12 and John 13:34. What do you think Jesus meant by "new command"? How has he asked you to trade in an interpretation of love limited by your own experiences for the audacious love of God for others?

4. Belinda discussed her need for *two* summits by quoting the Talmud: "We do not see things as they are. We see things as we are." She and Alyce each had to make clear decisions to summit their own personal mountains in order to catch a glimpse of God's perspective of who they were and are so they could see each other and the world the way God sees them. What mountain do you need to summit? What fears rise up in you as you stare at the steep path to the peak? What voices are telling you, "You are not enough"?

5. We physically and spiritually leave marks behind wherever we go. What thumbprints have been left on you by others? What thumbprints are you leaving on this world? On individuals? On yourself?

PART TWO: LEARNING TO LOVE

1. Belinda refers to the tilted room study, in which participants were challenged to find the "true upright" position while strapped to a tilted chair in a tilted room without windows or other clues as to how to orient. How does understanding our context help us orient ourselves to others? To ourselves? How does perspective-taking help us step imaginatively into the shoes of another person and use that understanding to guide our actions? How can learning to take another person's perspective be threatening to our own? How is it helpful? Describe how the physical, attributional, and conceptual attributes of perspective-taking increase your empathy awareness.

2. Think back to your empathy gap. What perspectives are you filling your gap with? Now think through how the three-step process—humanizing others, minding the gap, and shifting perspectives—helps you become brave enough to change the way you live and love through how you choose to bridge the gap.

3. After reading chapter five, what do you think Paul Tillich meant when he said in the chapter's beginning quote, "The first duty of love is to listen"? How is listening done with more than our ears? Why is empathetic listening different from simply hearing others? What challenges your ability to "listen into" instead of "listen at" others?

4. Listening is a skill hardwired into humans at birth and can be developed into empathetic listening with practice. Set aside time as an individual, partners, or a group to engage the empathy skills survey in appendix A, and then discuss as a group. What surprised you? Where do you want to change?

5. Read the section of the Sermon on the Mount in Luke 6:27-36. How did Jesus describe the actions of his children, or tribe? How can a tribe be both creative and destructive? What did Jesus indicate to his followers that made the difference?

6. Belinda suggests conflict is neither good nor bad, and it can become beneficial regardless of how we feel about conflict. It's what we *do* with it that makes the difference. What conflict are you walking through now that you hope will become a "beautiful collision"? What choices would you need to make to set your conflict on a different path?

7. Belinda says peacemaking is not entirely linear nor completely circular. It resides in the space between the spaces—the now and not yet of who we are and who we are becoming. How is our identity rooted in the way we deal with conflict? How does our identity grow with each conflict? How do conflicts change as we step more fully into our identity?

PART THREE: NOW, TAKE YOUR RISK

1. What are the "obstacle illusions" that prevent pursuing empathy as a spiritual practice? Have you experienced an inability to feel the pain of another? Have you ever felt someone else's pain too much? Have you had "empathy misses," those moments when you miss an opportunity to lean into empathy? What are they? What specific practices could you engage to decrease your misses and increase your empathy quotient?

2. Belinda discusses soul-efficacy, a skill geared toward helping us connect with challenging people in the context of difficult relationships. She believes we can successfully connect with others at a soul level of thoughts, feelings, and actions—in other words, believing we can connect helps us connect. Where do you need to increase your soul-efficacy? Remember, soul-efficacy is an act of empathetic faith. God stands at the ready to help you, if you just ask.

3. Empathy is a spiritual discipline we pursue within our power so we can do something beyond our power. What spiritual disciplines do you currently practice to help you embody love and compassion?

4. "Love is or it ain't. Thin love ain't love at all," wrote Toni Morrison. How are you dreaming for yourself or your community to grow more connected, avoiding apathy and indifference, and engaging sacrificial, embodied love? How can you practically take this dream to God, who the apostle Paul audaciously described as the one "who is able to do immeasurably more than all we ask or imagine, according to his power that is at work within us" (Ephesians 3:20)?

5. Belinda suggests that your thumbprint is a testimony to God's infinite, fractal-like image in you as well as a testimony to the image you form with others as the body of Christ. You are the soul-print of God. The actions we take when embodying empathy as a spiritual discipline root our faith in reality. How have you been marked by God so you can make his mark on others? You may find this question easier to answer by engaging the Empathy Diamond found in appendix B.

6. How can we think of empathy as worship to God? What does this look like in practice? How does empathy toward God affect our ability to take another's perspective? To listen empathetically? To step into conflict for the purpose of transforming it into opportunity? How did Jesus' worship embody empathy toward God? How do you?

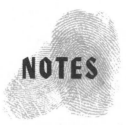

NOTES

PRELUDE

3   *Congo: The Worst Place:* "State of the World's Mothers Report 2013: Finland Best, Congo Worst," *Huffington Post*, May 7, 2013, www.huffingtonpost.com/2013 /05/07/state-of-the-worlds-mothers-report-2013_n_3224181.html.

INTRODUCTION

9   *levels of empathy:* Jamil Zaki, "What, Me Care? Young Are Less Empathetic," *Scientific American*, January 1, 2011, www.scientificamerican.com/article/what -me-care/.

Yet in a most recent study, only 40: Victor Lipman, "How Important Is Empathy to Successful Management?" *Forbes*, February 24, 2018, www.forbes.com /sites/victorlipman/2018/02/24/how-important-is-empathy-to-successful -management/#6a231f1ea46d.

empathy gap: Lipman, "How Important Is Empathy to Successful Management?"

apathy epidemic: Natasha Puri, "The Apathy Epidemic," *Huffington Post*, December 6, 2017, www.huffingtonpost.com/natasha-puri/the-apathy-epidemic _b_9797624.html.

10 *public shaming is on the rise:* See, for example, Mitch Albom, "The Ricochet Effect of Public Shaming Now on Full Display," *Detroit Free Press*, June 30, 2018, www.freep.com/story/sports/columnists/mitch-albom/2018/06/30 /mitch-albom-public-shaming/747998002/.

Americans are more divided: "Political Polarization in the American Public," 2014 Pew Research Study, www.people-press.org/2014/06/12/political -polarization-in-the-american-public/.

our malaise is not limited to politics: "NBC/WSJ Poll: Anger Defines 2016 Electorate," NBC News, September 27, 2015, www.nbcnews.com/meet-the-press /nbc-wsj-poll-anger-defines-2016-electorate-n435056.

Depression, a symptom of apathy, is now considered pandemic: Saptarshi Dutta, "1 in 20 People Suffer from Depression. It Is Time to Talk About This," Health Matters, January 5, 2018, https://sites.ndtv.com/healthmatters/1-in-20-people -suffer-from-depression-it-is-time-to-talk-about-this-1387/.

According to researchers of happiness and human flourishing: "How Empathy Can Change Your Life," infographic, Happify, www.happify.com/hd/empathy -can-change-your-life-infographic/?srid=hfp.

CHAPTER 1: BEAUTIFUL COLLISION

18 *I remember thinking:* portions of this section are from Belinda Bauman, "We Belong to Each Other," *Red Tent Living*, Nov. 9, 2017, https://redtentliving.com /2017/11/09/we-belong-to-each-other/.

19 *World Relief Congo:* World Relief has been empowering the local church to serve the most vulnerable for over seventy years. You can learn more about the program Odele and Esperance are a part of at worldrelief.org/conflict-zones.

20 *a woman as young as three:* Jeffery Gettleman, "Congo Study Sets Estimate for Rapes Much Higher," *New York Times*, May 12, 2011, www.nytimes.com /2011/05/12/world/africa/12congo.html.

The wars in this country: Vav Tampa, "Why the World Is Ignoring Congo War," CNN, November 27, 2012, www.cnn.com/2012/11/27/opinion/congo-war -ignored-vava-tampa/index.html.

22 *More than sixty million Americans:* Lydialyle Gibson, "The Nature of Loneliness," *University of Chicago Magazine,* November–December 2010, http:// magazine.uchicago.edu/1012/features/the-nature-of-loneliness.shtml.

23 *law of reciprocity:* "golden rule," Antony Flew, ed., *A Dictionary of Philosophy* (London: Pan Macmillan, 1979), 134.

Hurt not others in ways: "Priyavarga," Udānavarga 5:18 [139], www.ancient -buddhist-texts.net/Buddhist-Texts/S1-Udanavarga/05-Priya.htm.

What I do not wish men: Lun Yu, Analects 15:24, *The Analects* (English translation), James Legge, ed., Cambridge Chinese Classics, 48, www.camcc.org /_media/reading-group/lunyu/lunyu-en.pdf.

This is the sum of duty: Mahabharata 5:1517, *A Sourcebook for the Earth's Community of Religions* (Grand Rapids: CoNexus Press and New York: Global Education Associates, April 1995), 138.

to willfully and unjustly encroach: Harry J. Gensler, *Ethics and the Golden Rule: Do unto Others* (Oxford: Routledge, 2013), 35.

24 *We accept the love we think we deserve:* Stephen Chbosky, *The Perks of Being a Wallflower* (New York: Simon & Schuster, 1999), 24.

30 *the holiest object presented*: C. S. Lewis, *The Weight of Glory* (New York: Harper-One, 1980), 46.

CHAPTER 2: THE POWER OF EMPATHY

36 *I think the pursuit of happiness is the pursuit of reality:* Parker Palmer with Bill Moyers, "An Interview with Parker Palmer," transcript, PBS, February 20, 2009, www.pbs.org/moyers/journal/02202009/transcript2.html.

38   *We are tempted to think:* Sherry Turkle, "The Flight from Conversation," *New York Times*, April 21, 2012, www.nytimes.com/2012/04/22/opinion/sunday /the-flight-from-conversation.html.

40   *they are not alone:* Brené Brown, *Daring Greatly* (New York: Penguin Random House, 2012), 81.

   the art of stepping imaginatively: Roman Krznaric, "The Radical Power of Empathy," *Empathy: Why It Matters, and How to Get It* (New York: Penguin Random House, 2014), x.

46   *not simply wounded parties that need be compensated:* G. K. Chesterton, *On Lying in Bed and Other Essays* (Calgary: Bayeux Arts, 2000), 206.

48   *moving from neither understanding nor caring:* Personal class notes, "The Nature of Knowledge and Curriculum Integration," instructor Dr. William Davies, Covenant College, July 2012.

   His sister, Valentina, died: Belinda Bauman, "Life Forgotten, or Life Remembered? You Choose," *Red Tent Living*, March 14, 2018, https://redtentliving.com /2018/03/14/life-forgotten-or-life-remembered-you-choose/.

CHAPTER 3: MAKE YOUR MARK

59   *Take Leia, for example:* Leia Johnson is the founder and president of Somebody's Mama. After our Kilimanjaro adventure, she put her thoughts and wisdom to paper in a downloadable ebook called *Lectio*. All proceeds go to our partnership in ongoing projects helping women across the globe. Her work inspired me and gave me courage to write my own story. Find *Lectio* at www.somebodysmama.com.

62   *In a 1976 study, a group of Princeton Divinity School students:* J. M. Darley and C. D. Batson, "From Jerusalem to Jericho: A Study of Situational and Dispositional Variables in Helping Behavior," *Journal of Personality and Social Psychology* 1973, vol. 27, no. J, 100-8.

63   *It would seem that Our Lord:* C. S. Lewis, *The Weight of Glory* rev. ed. (New York: HarperCollins, 2001), 43, 257, 263-274.

71   *Here is our appeal to you:* Text of the 2014 Commencement address by Bill and Melinda Gates, *Stanford Report*, June 15, 2014, https://news.stanford.edu/news /2014/june/gates-commencement-remarks-061514.html.

CHAPTER 4: PERSPECTIVE-TAKING

76   *researchers Solomon Asch and H. A. Witkin:* Bill Reiche, "How Do You Know Which Way is Up?," *Popular Science*, December, 1950, 109-113.

77   *the art of stepping imaginatively:* Roman Krznaric, "The Radical Power of Empathy," *Empathy: Why It Matters, and How to Get It* (New York: Penguin Random House, 2014), x.

77   *theory of mind:* Lou Agosta, *Empathy Lessons* (Chicago: The Two Pears Press, 2018), 48-49.

79   *Learning life's lessons:* Elisabeth Kübler-Ross and David Kessler, *Life Lessons: Two Experts on Death and Dying Teach Us About the Mysteries of Life and Living* (New York: Scribner, 2000).

    Through others: Lev Vygotsky, "The Genesis of Higher Mental Functions," in R. Reiber, ed., *The History of the Development of Higher Mental Functions*, vol. 4 (New York: Plennum. 1987), 97-120.

81   *There's a communication chasm:* Mark Goulston and John Ullmen, *Real Influence: Persuade Without Pushing and Gain Without Giving In* (Nashville, TN: AMACOM, 2103).

82   *engaged selectively to simulate actions:* Katie Goldsmith, "The Social Brain," *Greater Good Magazine*, March 10, 2010, https://greatergood.berkeley.edu/article/item/the_social_brain.

85   *strengths, weaknesses, goals:* Mark Goulston and John Ullmen, "How to Really Understand Someone Else's Point of View," *Harvard Business Review*, April 22, 2013, https://hbr.org/2013/04/how-to-really-understand-someo.

CHAPTER 5: EMPATHETIC LISTENING

93   *Often when you're weary:* Austin Channing Brown, "Day 3 Devotional," in *Strength for the Climb: A Seven-Day Devotional Journey*, ed. Joy Beth Smith.

94   *The human race spends up to 80 percent:* "Hearing but Not Listening," USAF Aerospace Safety, January 1971, 8.

95   *I needed to hear those stories:* Portions of this section first appeared in Belinda Bauman, "Refugee Resettlement Isn't a Political Issue—It's a Humanitarian Issue," *Today's Christian Woman*, January 14, 2014, www.todayschristianwoman.com/articles/2014/january/to-see-and-be-seen.html.

96   *Congo is known as:* Belinda Bauman, "Congo's Superhero Moms," *The Daily Beast, Women in the World,* September 23, 2013.

101   *The art of conversation is being replaced:* Julian Treasure, "5 Ways to Listen Better," transcript, TED Talk, July 2011, www.ted.com/talks/julian_treasure_5_ways_to_listen_better?language=en.

102   *These little considerations for others:* Simon Sinek in Shelley Levitt, "Why the Empathetic Leader Is the Best Leader," *Success*, March 15, 2017, www.success.com/why-the-empathetic-leader-is-the-best-leader/.

    In cases of trauma: Joy Beth Smith, "Forgiving the Unforgivable? Shame, Silence and Sexual Abuse," *Today's Christian Woman,* March 30, 2016, www.todayschristianwoman.com/articles/2016/march-30/forgiving-unforgivable-sexual-abuse-allender.html.

103   *the hippocampus heals:* Smith, "Forgiving the Unforgivable?"

103   *If we share our story with someone:* Brené Brown, *Daring Greatly: How the Courage to Be Vulnerable Transforms the Way We Live, Love, Parent and Lead* (New York: Penguin Random House, 2012), 75.

104   *Half-eared listening:* Dietrich Bonhoeffer, *Life Together* (New York: Harper-Collins, 2015), 76.

108   *the story of the Rabbi and his son:* The story of the Rabbi and his son is first attributed to Rabbi Sholom DovBer Schneersohn and is found in many iterations.

CHAPTER 6: PEACEMAKING

114   *What! You too?:* C. S. Lewis, *The Four Loves* (New York: Harcourt, Brace, 1960), 65.

115   *Given this, it is no surprise:* Dr. Sanjay Gupta, "Why You Should Treat Loneliness as a Chronic Illness," Everyday Health, www.everydayhealth.com/news /loneliness-can-really-hurt-you/.

117   *Both were key to her survival:* This conversation is recorded as I remember it, but many of the more general details were informed by a documentary on the life of Elsie and Nicolas Hitimana. *Rwanda: Hope Rises* explores how Rwanda is healing and rebuilding in the aftermath of the 1994 genocide. Produced and directed by Trevor Meier, the full length movie can be purchased for screening at www.hoperisesfilm.com.

      Ikirezi: Ikirezi Natural Products is an emerging agribusiness pioneering the production of high quality essential oils in Rwanda. For more information, go to www.ikirezi.com.

119   *By the year 2000, 130,000 people:* Filip Reyntjens and Stef Vandeginste, "Rwanda: An Atypical Transition," in *Roads to Reconciliation*, eds. Elin Skaar, et al. (Lanham, MD: Lexington Books, 2005), 110.

120   *Conflicts between Rwandans:* "History," Gacaca Community Justice, 2018, http://gacaca.rw/about/history-3/.

      Judges and juries could try: Gitarama, "Judging Rawanda's Genocide: Justice on the Grass," *The Economist*, June 6, 2002, www.economist.com/middle-east -and-africa/2002/06/06/justice-on-the-grass.

124   *Wars can simmer at a low boil:* To learn more, read John Paul Lederach, *The Little Book of Conflict Transformation: Clear Articulation of the Guiding Principles by a Pioneer in the Field*, The Little Books of Justice and Peacebuilding Series (Intercourse, PA: Good Books, 2003).

125   *If we don't, we risk:* See Duane Elmer, *Cross-Cultural Servanthood: Serving the World in Christlike Humility* (Downers Grove, IL: InterVarsity Press, 2006).

127   *First, I am a Christian:* Personal conversation with Dina, May 2017; informed by an interview conducted by John Crosby, Christ Presbyterian Church, Edina,

Minnesota, July 2016, with Yohanna Katanacho, professor at Bethlehem Bible College, and Dina Katanacho, executive director of the Arab-Israeli Bible Society, www.cpconline.org/wp-content/uploads/2016/07/07-10-2016-Sermon -John-Crosby-Final.pdf.

129   *I couldn't see a face:* Leymah Gbowee with Carol Mithers, *Mighty Be Our Powers: How Sisterhood, Prayer, and Sex Changed a Nation at War: A Memoir* (New York: Beast, 2011), 140.

CHAPTER 7: OBSTACLE ILLUSIONS

136   *distorts our reasoning:* Paul Bloom, *Against Empathy: The Case for Rational Compassion* (New York: HarperCollins, 2016), 5.

  the biggest deficit that we have: Barack Obama in "Empathy Documentary, Barack Obama Promotes Empathy from Books and Literacy," August 27, 2010, www.youtube.com/watch?v=tg_qt_P8B40.

138   *drives people to treat others:* Bloom, *Against Empathy*, 30.

  Empathy is . . . a motivation to get us thinking: Denise Cummins, "Why Paul Bloom Is Wrong About Empathy and Morality," *Psychology Today*, October 20, 2013, www.psychologytoday.com/us/blog/good-thinking/201310/why-paul -bloom-is-wrong-about-empathy-and-morality.

139   *Cognitive empathy is a useful tool:* Bloom, *Against Empathy*, 233.

140   *over 30 percent of the American population:* Obsessive-Compulsive Disorder (OCD) Statistics, National Institute of Mental Health, November 2017, www .nimh.nih.gov/health/statistics/obsessive-compulsive-disorder-ocd.shtml.

147   *If you register empathy as a feeling:* Emiliana Simon-Thomas, "Is It Possible to Run Out of Empathy?," Hopes&Fears, 2015, www.hopesandfears.com/hopes/now /question/216857-is-it-possible-to-run-out-of-empathy.

  Find a way to connect: Simon-Thomas, "Is It Possible to Run Out of Empathy?"

148   *extreme state of tension:* Dr. Charles Figley, "Did You Know?," Compassion Fatigue Awareness Project, 2017, www.compassionfatigue.org/.

150   *Only if you feel or actively foster:* Stephanie D. Preston, "Is It Possible to Run Out of Empathy?," Hopes&Fears, 2015, www.hopesandfears.com/hopes/now /question/216857-is-it-possible-to-run-out-of-empathy.

CHAPTER 8: EMPATHY AS A SPIRITUAL DISCIPLINE

154   *the Telos group:* The Telos group envisions a world in which leaders and their communities claim the requisite drive, expertise, and relationships to effectively and relentlessly wage peace. You can learn more about them at www.telosgroup.org.

  In another part of Israel: Lynne Hybels's interview with parents at the Hand in Hand Center for Jewish-Arab Education in Israel (2015), www.handin handk12.org.

154 *One organization, Musalaha*: for more information, visit Musalaha, www
.musalaha.org/.

I AM PEACE Campaign: Paul Lorgerie, "Jerusalem High School Students Blow
a Peaceful Wind on Social Networks," *Palestine-Israel Journal*, July 7, 2015,
www.pij.org/details.php?blog=1&id=352.

155 *Tala Jean:* Personal interview with Tala Jean, May 2017.

Dallas Willard defined spiritual disciplines as: Dallas Willard, *The Spirit of the
Disciplines: Understanding How God Changes Lives* (San Francisco: Harper-
Collins, 1991), 156.

156 *Quoting James S. Stewart, Willard:* Willard, *The Spirit of the Disciplines*, 96.

157 *Trappist monk and activist Thomas Merton:* Thomas Merton, *Contemplation in
a World of Action*, 2nd ed. (Norte Dame, IN: University of Notre Dame Press,
1998), 160-61.

Make sure that [the prayers]: C. S. Lewis, *The Screwtape Letters* (New York:
Harper Collins, 1943), 12.

158 *We must not be led:* Richard J. Foster, *Celebration of Discipline: The Path to
Spiritual Growth* (San Francisco: HarperCollins, 1998), 1-2.

this and that: Michael Metzger, "This and That," Clapham Institute, April 9,
2018, www.doggieheadtilt.com/this-and-that.

159 *Willpower will never succeed in dealing:* Foster, *Celebration of Discipline*, 5.

161 *with the ability to become anyone or anything:* Dr. Martha Beck, "Have a Heart:
The Empathy Workout," *Oprah Magazine*, March 2006, www.oprah.com
/spirit/martha-beck-have-a-heart/all.

164 *Now imitate, as closely as you:* Beck, "Have a Heart."

165 *Highly empathetic people:* Roman Krznaric, "Six Habits of Highly Empathic
People," *Greater Good Magazine*, November 27, 2012, https://greatergood
.berkeley.edu/article/item/six_habits_of_highly_empathic_people1.

167 *The most beautiful people I have known:* Elisabeth Kübler-Ross, *Death: The Final
Stage of Growth* (New York: Touchstone, 1975), 93.

CHAPTER 9: THE THUMBPRINT OF GOD

174 *Order doesn't come by itself:* Benoit Mandelbrot, "A Theory of Roughness: A Talk
with Benoit Mandelbrot," Edge, December 20, 2004, www.edge.org/3rd_culture
/mandelbrot04/mandelbrot04_index.html.

176 *the #MeToo and #ChurchToo movements captured:* The #MeToo movement was
founded by civil rights activist and community organizer Tarana Burke. The
#ChurchToo movement was cofounded by spoken-word artist Emily Joy and
author Hannah Paasch.

178   *SheLoves Magazine:* The mission of *SheLoves Magazine* is to mobilize and empower women, so we may transform our world together. Learn more at shelovesmagazine.com/about.

178   *[The video] shook me:* Idelette McVicker, "Our Indigenous Sisters are Sacred," *SheLoves Magazine*, March 7, 2018, http://shelovesmagazine.com/2018/indigenous-sisters-sacred.

179   *While it's difficult to identify:* Brenna, "Violent Victimization."

    indigenous women are three and half times: Shannon Brenna, "Violent Victimization of Aboriginal Women in the Canadian Provinces, 2009," *Juristat*, 2011, www.statcan.gc.ca/pub/85-002-x/2011001/article/11439-eng.htm.

    A part of us will always be missing: McVicker, "Our Indigenous Sisters are Sacred."

183   *Well over 70 percent:* William Spindler, "Survey Finds Syrian Refugees in Lebanon Became Poorer, More Vulnerable in 2017," United Nations High Commission on Refugees, January 9, 2018, www.unhcr.org/en-us/news/briefing/2018/1/5a548d174/survey-finds-syrian-refugees-lebanon-poorer-vulnerable-2017.html.

185   *According to the United Nations:* Operational Portal, Syria Regional Refugee Response, United Nations High Commission on Refugees, accessed October 10, 2018, https://data2.unhcr.org/en/situations/syria.

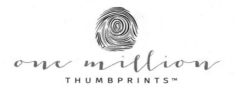

ONE MILLION
THUMBPRINTS™

THE MANDATE

To build a global movement of peacemakers who are dedicated to overcoming the devastating effects of war on women.

THE PROBLEM

Every day, millions of women experience brutal violence as a result of conflict and war. In Congo alone, seven out of ten women have experienced sexual violence. And yet these cases continue to be underreported. Female victims of war continue to be forgotten, silenced, and excluded from efforts to rebuild, despite their ability to assist in recovery and take on leadership roles in peace-building efforts.

THE CAMPAIGN

One Million Thumbprints is dedicated to fostering resilience and dignity in the lives of these brave women. The campaign takes on a two-pronged approach: advocating for the vigorous implementation of policy that will help protect women in conflict zones and partnering with organizations that are already on the ground meeting practical needs, including food, clothing, shelter, and trauma assistance.

THE INVITATION

When Esperance asked Belinda to "tell the world" her story, she signed her request with a thumbprint. Her thumbprint became our mandate: *Violence against her is violence against us.* Each thumbprint collected for 1MT is a visual representation of solidarity, but it's also a call to action.

THE CLIMBS

The peacemakers of 1MT actively seek to embody empathy with their suffering sisters and to honor their strength. We decide what high ground we will summit—be it a hill or a mountain—and climb with our sisters in our minds and hearts. We raise our banners of thumbprints in honor of the brave souls we fight for worldwide. We climb united with these women to bring the violent acts committed against them into light through advocacy, storytelling, and fundraising.

JOIN US

Twitter: @OneMT
Facebook: One Million Thumbprints
Instagram: @onemillionthumbprints
Web: www.onemillionthumbprints.org

Mail: One Million Thumbprints
PO Box 230132
Grand Rapids, MI 49523
Text "thumbprint" to 51555